Trauma-Responsive Family Engagement in Early Childhood

Designed for all professionals working with parents and families of young children, this practical guide offers comprehensive resources for building trauma-responsive family engagement in your school or program. Throughout this book, you'll find:

- ♦ Evidence-based practices that promote trauma-responsive family engagement.
- ♦ Exercises and tools for identifying the strengths and learning edges within your program, school, or agency.
- ♦ Vignettes from people and programs striving to create trusting, asset-focused partnerships with families that improve equity and promote culturally responsive practices.
- ♦ Reflective inquiry questions and sample conversations to help you examine your own practices.

With concrete examples and easy-to-implement strategies, this critical book helps readers put theory into practice while providing essential support for individuals and groups both new to and experienced with trauma-responsive practices in early childhood.

Julie Nicholson is Professor of Practice in the School of Education at Mills College and Co-Director of the Center for Equity in Early Childhood Education.

Julie Kurtz is CEO at the Center for Optimal Brain Integration® and trains on social-emotional and trauma-responsive practices across the lifespan. She also operates a private practice as a licensed marriage and family therapist in California, USA.

Other Eye On Education Books

Available From Routledge
(www.routledge.com/k-12)

**Creating Inclusive Writing Environments in the K-12
Classroom: Reluctance, Resistance, and Strategies
that Make a Difference**
Angela Stockman

**Trauma-Informed Practices for Early Childhood Educators:
Relationship-Based Approaches that support Healing
and Build Resilience in Young Children**
Julie Nicholson, Linda Perez, and Julie Kurtz

**Culturally Responsive Self-Care Practices for Early
Childhood Educators**
Julie Nicholson, Priya Shimpi Driscoll, Julie Kurtz,
Doménica Márquez, and LaWanda Wesley

**Implementing Project Based Learning in Early
Childhood: Overcoming Misconceptions
and Reaching Success**
Sara Lev, Amanda Clark, and Erin Starkey

**Advocacy for Early Childhood Educators: Speaking Up for
Your Students, Your Colleagues, and Yourself**
Colleen Schmit

**Grit, Resilience, and Motivation in Early Childhood:
Practical Takeaways for Teachers**
Lisa B. Fiore

**Trauma-Responsive Practices for Early Childhood
Leaders: Creating and Sustaining Healing Engaged
Organizations**
Julie Nicholson, Julie Kurtz, Jen Leland, Lawanda Wesley,
and Sarah Nadiv

Trauma-Responsive Family Engagement in Early Childhood

Practices for Equity and Resilience

Julie Nicholson and Julie Kurtz
with Laura Rivas, Tasha Henneman,
Eric Peterson, Shawn Bryant, and Betty Lin

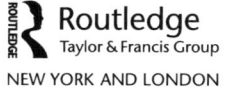

Routledge
Taylor & Francis Group

NEW YORK AND LONDON

First published 2022
by Routledge
605 Third Avenue, New York, NY 10158

and by Routledge
2 Park Square, Milton Park, Abingdon, Oxon OX14 4RN

Routledge is an imprint of the Taylor & Francis Group, an informa business

© 2022 Julie Nicholson and Julie Kurtz

Library of Congress Cataloging-in-Publication Data
A catalog record for this title has been requested

ISBN: 978-0-367-65065-0 (hbk)
ISBN: 978-0-367-64701-8 (pbk)
ISBN: 978-1-003-12766-6 (ebk)

DOI: 10.4324/9781003127666

Typeset in Palatino
by Newgen Publishing UK

Contents

Meet the Authors

Julie Nicholson is Professor of Practice in the School of Education at Mills College and Co-Director of the Center for Equity in Early Childhood Education.

Julie Kurtz is CEO at the Center for Optimal Brain Integration® and trains on social-emotional and trauma-responsive practices across the lifespan. She also operates a private practice as a licensed marriage and family therapist in California, USA.

Laura Rivas is a Family Engagement Specialist for the Berkeley Unified School District.

Tasha Henneman is Chief of Government and Policy for the Positive Resources Center.

Eric Peterson is Director—Client Services and Public Policy, BANANAS Resource and Referral Agency.

Shawn Bryant is Founding Director and Chief Learning Officer Teaching Excellence Center.

Betty Lin is Program Coordinator, Elementary and Autism Programs, Alameda Unified School District.

Introduction: An Urgent Need for Trauma-Sensitive Family Engagement Practices in Early Childhood

Young children and their parents and family members are increasingly impacted by a wide range of daily stressors and traumatic experiences. Racism, poverty, housing and food insecurity, loss of employment, distress related to immigration, migration and/or deportation, natural disasters, community violence, child maltreatment and intimate partner violence, health concerns and lack of access to medical care are just some of the factors impacting families today and creating an urgent need for trauma-responsive early childhood environments. Adult caregivers struggling with their own stress and trauma can unknowingly and unintentionally increase children's perceptions of danger and threat. As children are impacted by the emotional state of their caregivers, stress activation in adults has an immediate and harmful impact on children's vulnerable and developing brains and bodies by starting a cascade of physiological responses that can impair their learning and development throughout their lifespan. If, however, adults have access to relationships and

DOI: 10.4324/9781003127666-1

environments that reduce their stress and support their ability to cope and heal, they are less likely to negatively impact the young children in their care.

Early childhood professionals are in a unique position to partner with parents and family members to strengthen their ability to cope through adversity (building resilience). In building resilience there are positive impacts such as reducing stress for young children and preventing the short and long-term impact of toxic stress and trauma from derailing their ability to learn, develop and thrive to their optimal potential. Trauma-responsive family engagement supports early childhood professionals to:

◆ Create trusting relationships with families rooted in empathy and a responsiveness to their diverse lived experiences and hopes and dreams for their children

◆ Strengthen their knowledge of and capacity to use co-regulation and attunement strategies to prevent and/or disrupt harmful and deficit-based interactions with parents and families

◆ Develop genuine power-sharing partnerships with families that strengthens trust and dismantles sources of distrust based in historical trauma and cycles of oppression

◆ Build parents' and families' resilience, coping skills and pathways to healing

It is an unfortunate reality that an increasing number of young children and their families are entering early learning programs having experienced trauma or living in conditions of toxic stress (Bethell, Davis, Gombojav, Stumbo & Powers, 2017). As a result, there is an ever present need to increase our individual and collective understanding of how to build relationships, communicate and work with parents and family members in a trauma-sensitive manner that not only reduces stress and prevents harm and re-traumatization, but also strengthens adults' and children's capacity for joy, resilience, health and well-being. The time is now to implement trauma-responsive resilience building and healing centered family engagement practices throughout the early childhood field.

This book complements our first three books—*Trauma-Informed Practices for Early Childhood Educators: Relationship-Based Approaches that Support Healing and Build Protective Factors in Young Children* (2019), *Culturally Responsive Self-Care for Early Childhood Educators* (2020) and *Trauma Responsive Practices for Early Childhood Leaders: Creating and Sustaining Healing Engaged Organizations* (2021)—by considering how an understanding of trauma, resilience, equity and healing centered practices can be integrated into a respectful, responsive and attuned approach to family engagement.

What Is Family Engagement?

Family Engagement has been defined in a variety of ways by different scholars, clinicians and agencies. We highlight three below that inspire our work:

> Family engagement is an interactive process through which program staff and families, family members, and their children build positive and goal-oriented relationships. It is a shared responsibility of families and professionals that requires mutual respect for the roles and strengths each has to offer. Family engagement means doing with—not doing to or for—families. At the program level, family engagement involves parents' engagement with their children and with staff as they work together toward the goals that families choose for themselves and their children. It also involves families and staff working toward goals to improve the program. Head Start and Early Head Start staff work together with families, other professionals, and community partners in ways that promote equity, inclusiveness, and cultural and linguistic responsiveness.
>
> (U.S. Department of Health and Human Services, 2018, p. 2)

Family engagement is a shared responsibility among providers, caregivers, and families in which institutions and organizations commit to working with families in meaningful and culturally respectful ways. Family engagement is continuous across a child's life from cradle to career and carried out everywhere children learn—at home, in childcare settings, in health settings, and in community places and spaces.

(National Association for Family, School, and Community Engagement Policy Council, 2010)

A third definition emerging in critical family engagement research and advocacy rooted in anti-racist and community organizing explicitly privileges parents and family members as experts with valuable insight on educational reform efforts including work to transform and improve schools and school systems (Ishimaru, Lott, Torres & O-Reilly-Diaz, 2019). Parents and family members are positioned as powerful change agents who can advocate on behalf of their children, intervene and inform adaptations to educational policies and practices, resist and remove barriers to education and work in solidarity with larger movements for intersectional justice faced by historically marginalized families and communities (Baquedano-López, Alexander & Hernandez, 2013).

Making It Real. In the Daily Life of One Early Childhood Professional, Family Engagement Is…

♦ Understanding that family engagement happens from the first point of contact

♦ Knowing that I can't be effective in my work with a child unless I understand the context and conditions where the child comes from…which is their family

♦ Disrupting any deficit-based language, stories and assumptions about parents and families I work with and instead, finding the strengths and capacity that each family has and using that knowledge to build our program and move it forward

◆ Listening to, and actually valuing, what families are saying to me even if it is not a value that I hold. Embracing the fundamental belief that my morals and values may not be the family's morals and values and this difference does not equate to deficit

◆ Finding out what a family's needs are

◆ Keeping my program's policies and procedures fluid, responsive and flexible to a new group of entering families

◆ Co-creating experiences with families that are meaningful to them

◆ Communicating and requesting information from families in a way that allows them to feel safe and to have a sense of agency and control in how the information is used and/or shared

◆ Acknowledging that every interaction either builds trust or degrades trust and that many small interactions help families to feel safe and are the glue to building trust

◆ Recognizing the power differential in my communication with families. Striving to share power "with" parents vs. having power "over" them. This means limiting or avoiding the use of jargon, lecturing and/or telling them what to do

◆ Reminding myself that behavior I perceive to be challenging or difficult is rooted in families' care and concern about their child and their outcomes

◆ Having conversations that are meaningful to the family. This means, in every interaction, linking and building on what is of interest to the family; a practice that strengthens trust, attunement and partnerships

◆ Being thankful that a family is asking me a question about the program or my approach in caring for their child

◆ Communicating messages and supporting families to feel like they are "doing enough"

◆ Spotlighting everyday interactions (everyday routines/ activities with their child) that reflect what families are doing well and using these as opportunities to spotlight or teach and learn in the context of relationships (e.g., during the ride to preschool on the bus, train, or car they can discuss what will happen at school. Discussing what's about to happen is a successful strategy to support children who may have experienced direct or secondary trauma)

◆ Having classroom environments and activities that represent and respect the family's culture and language

◆ Giving families opportunities to share their ideas, opinions and feedback free of judgment. Not always doing what is on *our* checklist, but also including what is on the family's checklist, that is, what is meaningful to them

◆ Taking time to slow down, connect and reflect with families versus being in a hurry

◆ Recognizing that families are trusting us with their precious child

◆ Noticing how families are feeling, understanding and responding to what's been said, presented, or what happened in our program

◆ Shifting and asking families if we can come to their community tables (church, community center, mosque); all the places families live and exist

◆ Acting as allies supporting families in their own decisions

◆ Understanding that in early childhood and family services, racism and inequity has often presented itself as "help" or support based in deficit thinking (e.g., describing achievement or opportunity gaps, or children's "lack" of readiness for kindergarten versus thinking about readiness for schools, teachers, families and communities)

◆ A path to equitable education and community-based opportunities for families

◆ Should be a #1 priority to create more equitable opportunities to involve and engage families, give families power, voice and control in their child's care and
education.

(Shawn M. Bryant, Founding Director and Chief
Learning Officer at Teaching Excellence Center)

What Does the Research Say About Family Engagement?

Decades of research provides consistent evidence that positive,
respectful and mutually trusting relationships between families and early learning programs and schools is associated with
many benefits for young children, for families and for the early
childhood field. A sample of these research findings includes:

◆ Families' knowledge, skills, cultural assets, routines and
practices create the foundations for supporting young
children's development, positive life outcomes and
family well-being (NCPFCE, 2014; National Research
Council and Institute of Medicine, 2000).

◆ Parent/family-child relationships and family well-being
are strongly associated with young children's long-term
development across domains (cognitive, social emotional,
physical), learning trajectories, social experiences, health
and well-being (Anda et al., 2006; National Research
Council and Institute of Medicine, 2000).

◆ When families have strong social supports with peers
and access to comprehensive services and community
resources they value and need, children are happier
and have better short and long-term health outcomes
(National Academies of Sciences, Engineering, and
Medicine, 2015; NCPFCE, 2013).

◆ Non-dominant families—e.g., those who are traditionally marginalized and minoritzed[1] including Black,
Indigenous and People of Color—can become powerful

actors in equity-based educational change when issues of power, race, culture, language and class are integrated into family engagement efforts (Baquedano-López et al., 2013; Cooper, 2009; Ippolito, 2015; Ishimaru, 2014a; 2014b; 2017; Ishimaru, Lott, Torres & Diaz, 2019; Mediratta, Shah & McAlister, 2009; Olivos, 2006; Warren, Hong, Rubin & Uy, 2009; Warren, Mapp, and The Community Organizing and School Reform Project, 2011).

◆ Effective family engagement is most likely to emerge in early childhood programs that value and strive to create power-sharing partnerships based in relational trust with families, where communication is based in open, ongoing, two-way communication (Reedy & McGrath, 2010, USDHHS, 2018).

◆ Early childhood professionals' positive experiences with family engagement enhance their professional learning and job satisfaction (Holochwost, DeMott, Buell, Yannetta & Amsden, 2009; Wells, 2015).

Trauma Informed versus Trauma Responsive

To be informed is to receive information. To be transformed is to be changed or altered as a result of this new knowledge.

—Brandt (2020)

Although the more familiar and commonly used term in research, professional literature and professional development is "trauma informed," we have opted to primarily use the term "trauma responsive" throughout this book. We believe that building awareness of trauma and its impact and trauma-sensitive family engagement strategies to become *trauma informed*, is an essential first step, but not sufficient. Instead, we advocate for going beyond a process of building awareness and understanding towards applying this knowledge in practice. **To be *trauma responsive* is to take actions for positive change**, to use knowledge of trauma and resilience to make changes to language and beliefs, to critically examine and revise policies and to make shifts to practices with both the children and families. To be trauma responsive is therefore, to be trauma informed, however, the reverse is not necessarily true. Looking at trauma-responsive family engagement, we must aspire as Shawn Bryant says to "move from practices that are solely child-centered to involving and engaging families from the first phone call they make to enroll in our programs."

Balancing a Focus on Trauma with Coping, Resilience and Healing

It is essential to balance any discussion of trauma with an equal if not more robust naming of strengths, coping, resilience and healing. No individual, family, community, cultural group or organization wants to be defined by their vulnerabilities and the bad things that happen to them (Ginwright, 2018) and focusing solely on peoples' vulnerabilities and traumatic experiences can perpetuate cycles of trauma and oppression. In contrast, when stories of stress and trauma are honestly acknowledged but balanced with discussions of coping, strengths and resilience we create the conditions to buffer stress, prevent negative impacts from trauma and support healing.

We draw on Dr. Shawn Ginwright's discussion of healing centered engagement. Dr. Ginwright, author of *Hope and Healing in Urban Education: How Activists are Reclaiming Matters of the Heart* and *The Future of Healing: Shifting From Trauma Informed Care to Healing Centered Engagement* (2018), explains that although the idea of trauma-informed approaches in education is important, he believes it is incomplete. He states this is the case for several reasons:

♦ Trauma-informed education correctly highlights the specific needs for individuals who have exposure to trauma but incorrectly assumes that all trauma is an individual experience rather than a collective one
♦ Our current focus on trauma-informed approaches in education does not address the root causes of trauma in

neighborhoods, families, and schools. And because trauma is a collective experience in many cases, we need to disrupt the environmental contexts (the toxic systems, policies and practices) that caused the harm in the first place

◆ Instead of emphasizing the experience and impact of trauma we need to spend more time fostering healing and strengthening the roots of well-being

Dr. Ginwright advocates for a more holistic approach and a wider a range of healing centered options—inspired by the fields of positive psychology and community psychology—for responding to trauma and fostering well-being. This approach shifts the focus from a treatment-based model which views trauma and harm as an isolated experience to an engagement model which is strengths-based, emphasizes a collective view of healing and re-centers culture and identity/intersectional justice as central aspects of well-being. Additionally, a healing centered approach acknowledges that well-being comes from participating in transforming the underlying causes of harm within our societal structures and institutions.

Resilience as a Balance Scale

We also draw from and adapt Harvard's Center on the Developing Child's description of resilience as a balance scale in the lives of adults and children.

On one side of the scale are parents' and families' **negative experiences that tip the scale toward unhealthy levels of stress, trauma and harm.** Examples of the negative stressors that impact many parents and families in early childhood programs:

◆ Discrimination and racism
◆ Housing and/or food insecurity and insufficiency
◆ Unemployment, job loss
◆ Physical or mental health concerns
◆ Isolation/lack of support
◆ Difficulty in relationships
◆ Struggle to keep up with expenses

◆ Symptoms of anxiety or depression
◆ Lack of health insurance and/or lower-quality physical and mental health treatment
◆ Barriers preventing access to social safety net services (e.g., discrimination in employment or housing policies)
◆ Fewer economic buffers during periods of hardship

When children and adults have exposure to **multiple, simultaneous, or long-lasting hardships** they are at greater risk for having short and long-term consequences. The accumulation of multiple stressors can overwhelm even the most resilient individuals and make it difficult for them to access their social, emotional, psychological and spiritual forms of coping, resilience and healing. It is important for early childhood professionals to understand that Latinx, Black and Native American low-income families experience multiple hardships at greater rates than Asian and White low-income families. Racial and ethnic disparities in the number and co-occurrence of multiple hardships/

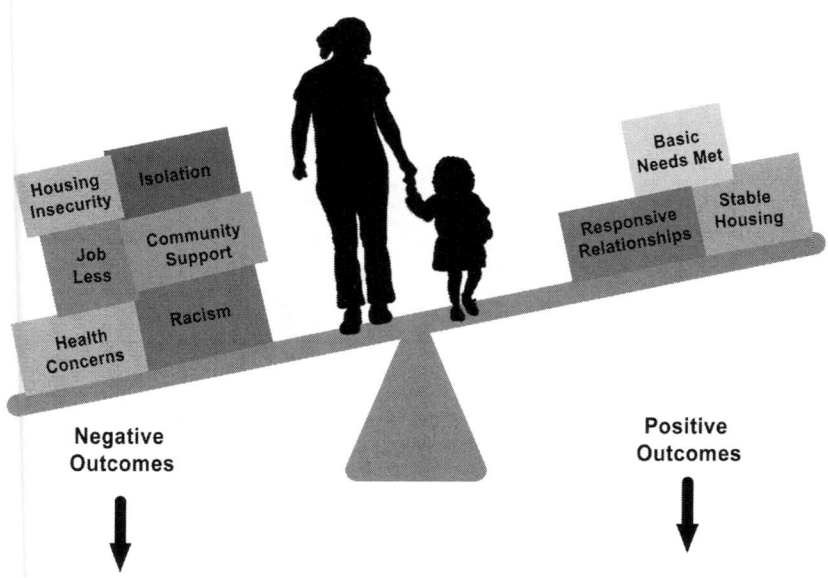

FIGURE 0.1
Negative Balance Scale
Source: Alice Blecker. Graphic adapted from original source: https://developingchild. harvard.edu/resources/inbrief- the- science-of-resilience/

adversities is a reflection of the inequities embedded in our nation's structures (housing, education, criminal justice, labor, finance, etc.) and institutions (agencies, programs, schools) and the policies that have historically and continue to make it difficult for these families to achieve economic stability and to have access to economic buffers during periods of hardship (e.g., job loss, medical emergency, homelessness; Kendi, 2019; Padilla & Thomson, 2021).

> Latino and Black families are less likely to have economic buffers during periods of hardship. This is primarily due to systemic factors, like discrimination in housing policies, that limit Black homeownership and to systems that perpetuate racial/ethnic gaps in wealth distribution, such as inheritances and university legacy policies, which overwhelmingly benefit those with White parents. Discrimination contributes to the tendency for Hispanic and Black individuals to receive less and lower-quality physical and mental health treatment and to experience greater barriers to accessing social safety net services. … it is much more likely that Hispanic and Black families will experience not just a single, temporary stressor, but an accumulation of multiple hardships …while most children are resilient in the face of singular or time-limited stressors, especially when supported by sensitive and responsive caregivers, exposure to multiple, simultaneous, or long-lasting hardships may potentially overwhelm a child's stress-response system. This, in turn, can impact their attention and regulation of emotion, with the potential for detrimental effects on their learning, behavior, and health. This accumulation of stressors can also overwhelm adults' psychological resources, making government resources more important than ever—especially those that help parents remain economically afloat and able to financially and psychologically support their children in times of hardship.
>
> (Padilla & Thomson, 2021)

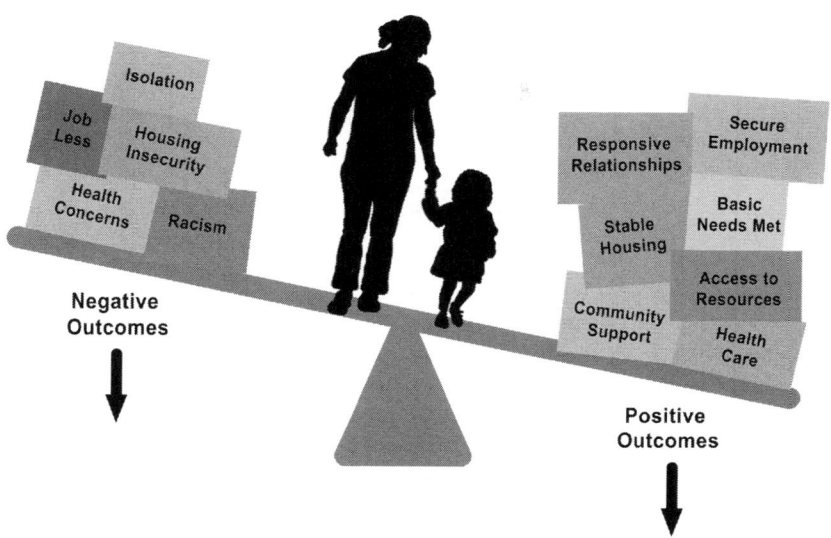

FIGURE 0.2
Positive Balance Scale
Source: Alice Blecker

On the other side of the scale are the **positive experiences and resilience factors that tip the scale toward coping, health, wellness and positive outcomes**. Positive experiences reduce stress and vulnerability for parents and families and strengthen their ability to cope, heal and thrive. Examples of positive experiences include consistent and caring responsive relationships, having basic living needs met (financial, housing, food, clothing), feeling a sense of belonging and inclusion and access to resources.

   Resilience factors can be both **internal** and/or **external**. **Internal resilience** is "built into our wiring" such as the temperament we are born with. **External resilience** is learned (taking a class on child development) or when we have access to resources (community supports, food, housing shelter, childcare). Both internal and external resilience factors can protect us from stress. Understanding the factors that will help families tip the scale in the positive direction is critical to trauma-responsive family engagement.

Internal resilience factors including	External resilience factors including
Temperament traits	Learning a new skill (taking a class on child development, listening to a podcast, reading a book)
Outlook on life (positive or idealistic to realistic/constructive)	Access to meet basic needs (food, housing, clothing)
Activity or energy levels (high to low)	Access to community supports (food pantry, childcare)
Sensitivity (tolerance for external stimulus such as sounds, smells, temperature, touch, taste)	Being a part of a community (book club, parent class, spiritual community, running group)
Adaptability (tolerance for uncertainty, change, transitions, new information)	Helping others

The center of the scale is the **"fulcrum" which can shift its placement across a person's lifespan** based on their life experiences. Over time, if an individual or family has many positive life experiences and develops a range of coping skills, the fulcrum will shift its position making it easier to enjoy health, wellness and to achieve positive outcomes. In contrast, the cumulative effect of many negative experiences can be a shift of the fulcrum to the left making the individual or family more vulnerable to stress, trauma and negative outcomes. Each person's and each individual family's stress/resilience scale will look different as we respond to stress in unique ways based on a range of factors (e.g., neurobiology, history of trauma, access to support, etc.). Our perceptions of stress change throughout the day so the balance of our individual scales is dynamic and responsive to the changing conditions in our daily lives.

Many families we work with are experiencing stress, high cumulative risk factors or have trauma histories—all of which compound to impact their resilience/stress scale. Often parents and families with young children have scales that are weighted to the side of stress. What can you as an individual or program do to buffer families' toxic stress, to lighten their negative load and to promote their coping and resilience? We can support families to tip their scales to the positive side of the resilience scale by promoting positive experiences—especially through nurturing and **responsive relationships**. The one thing that most children who develop resilience have in common is a stable, committed relationship with a supportive parent, caregiver or other adult. Adults need those supportive relationships, too! Other ways you can support parents and families to shift their scale's fulcrum to the right side of the scale include:

- ◆ Supporting families to meet basic living needs such as connecting them with community resources and programs that can help provide them with access food, shelter, diapers, health care, child care, rent and internet access
- ◆ Providing support or resources in times of need (i.e., loss, death, natural disaster, health concern, transitions)
- ◆ Ensuring communication is in multiple languages and that communication is offered in multiple formats (in person, via phone calls, text messages or video chats, written communication and at drop off or pick up) and in language that is accessible. Remembering that you're not just sharing information; you're also providing parents with time to engage in a responsive relationship
- ◆ Sharing positive experiences or interactions about their child on a regular basis
- ◆ Providing training and access to community support groups
- ◆ Creating opportunities for families to network and build social connections with other families
- ◆ Providing safe and predictable environments for families when they come to the program
- ◆ Ensuring the environment and materials in the classroom represent the families' cultural background
- ◆ Taking time to listen and to include the voices of families in policy and program development. Also, providing formal and informal opportunities for families to provide input, to voice their concerns and/or file a grievance

Articulating Your "Why" for Trauma-Responsive Family Engagement

> My "why" is simply that every time I have attempted to work with young children by themselves, I'm unsuccessful. When I have positioned the work with young children in the context and conditions of their family, my success rate grew. So it was my own firsthand experiences that taught me the importance of being family-centered. I think that one of the ways we can create more equitable school opportunities is to engage families from the very beginning, from their first call when they say, "I want to enroll my child." These are crucial moments that we can help them feel, "Oh, this school is valuing me and my child." Not just, "here's how you need to sign in and sign out, if you're late, this is how much the fee is." Family engagement gives families the opportunity to have control and have a voice in what they and their child are learning. How powerful is that?
>
> (Shawn M. Bryant, Founding Director & Chief Learning Officer at Teaching Excellence Center)

Understanding and clearly communicating your program or school's rationale—your "WHY"—for embarking on the journey to implement trauma responsive and healing centered family engagement is essential. This work is difficult and requires a long-term commitment. It can only be sustained when staff at all levels understand and are committed to the values, mission and vision driving the work. It's easy to fall into a trap of focusing on the *what* (content) and the *how* (operations and implementation). While these are important, this work can only be successful and sustainable if people take time to identify the "whys" that will fuel their passion, effort, investment and commitment to become trauma responsive and healing centered in work with families.

As Authors, What Is Driving Our Purpose and Passion Is to Imagine a Future Where Trauma- Responsive Healing Centered Family Engagement Is a Central Element of Early Childhood Programs and Services

We want every parent and family participating in early childhood programs and services to have access and opportunities to experience:

♦ Consistent, trusting, attuned and caring relationships
♦ A felt sense of belonging, dignity, worth and affirmation of their strengths, identities and cultural assets and ways of being and knowing
♦ Respect for the unique and diverse ideas, voices, values, perceptions, beliefs and cultural perspectives that they bring into our programs and *to be seen and heard*
♦ Opportunities for agency and control (voice and choice) including diverse choices and pathways to be involved and engaged
♦ A felt sense of safety and protection from the systems, structures, policies and people that cause harm. And when harm does occur…
♦ Allyship in disrupting inequity/harms in addition to have support to cope, build resilience, repair and heal

Reflection/Discussion Questions

Each program, school and community will have their own "why" that is rooted in your local histories, people and relationships, contexts and conditions.

♦ List one way in which you involve or engage families. Now can you think of "why" or the intention (e.g., value, cultural belief, mission, desired change or outcome) that inspires this practice?

◆ Can you think of one way in which you have given a family a voice in your early childhood program? Can you list one or more reasons "why" you provided this family an opportunity to have a voice?

As a field, we have always had parents and family members of infants, toddlers and preschool aged children entering the doors of our programs with many experiences of toxic stress and trauma including, but not limited to, homelessness, migration-immigration or deportation stress, community violence, domestic abuse, racism, poverty and natural disasters (fires, earthquakes, hurricanes and our current coronavirus pandemic). The current hardships, conditions of uncertainty, sudden illness, profound losses and deaths resulting from the coronavirus impacting families around the world, are exacerbating individual and collective experiences of toxic stress and trauma. The unprecedented nature of these conditions means that more than ever, our early educators, administrators and system leaders have urgency to communicate and interact with parents and families using a trauma-responsive and resilience building approach.

Although many important resources currently exist to describe effective family engagement practices for early learning environments (Berger & Riojas-Cortez, 2020; Grant & Ray, 2019; Muhs, 2019), there are currently no books available in our field that integrate the neuroscience of stress and trauma with a discussion of high quality family engagement practices. In fact, the only discussion of trauma in current publications is often limited to chapters on family violence and child abuse, reporting requirements for educators and characteristics of abusive parents. Our approach is quite different. We contend that although trauma-responsive approaches are essential for our work with parents and families impacted by trauma, they are also beneficial and improve our communication and engagement with all adults and children.

Unique Features of This Book

Everything in this book is written explicitly for the early childhood workforce. That is, all professionals who are working directly with, or on behalf of, parents and family members of infants, toddlers, preschoolers and early elementary-aged children including:

- ◆ Prospective, new to the field, as well as veteran early childhood educators working with young children (birth-8) in a range of contexts (family childcare, private and state subsidized centers, home visitation, foster families, community playgroups etc.)
- ◆ Family engagement specialists, coaches, professional development training and technical assistance staff
- ◆ Home visitors and mental health specialists
- ◆ Non-profit leaders, site supervisors, program directors, infrastructure staff and individuals working in state or federal early childhood policy or quality improvement and/or systems building initiatives
- ◆ Elementary school principals, Chief Academic Officers and other district administrators and support personnel with backgrounds outside early childhood who are increasingly being asked to support and work with early childhood educators
- ◆ Community college and university faculty and child and family researchers
- ◆ Funders

Throughout the book we include rich vignettes and case examples that provide many windows into examples of trauma-responsive family engagement practices in early childhood programs, schools and organizations. We share honest and authentic narratives—reported from early childhood professionals working in diverse contexts committed to this work—that acknowledge their strengths, small wins and progress as well as the many barriers they face and the different

Note

1 **Minoritized.** "A social group that is devalued in society. The devaluing encompasses how the group is represented, what degree of access to resources is granted, and how the unequal access is rationalized. The term *minoritized* (rather than minority) is used to indicate that the group's lower position is a function of active socially constructed dynamics, rather than its numbers in society" (DiAngelo, 2016, p. 61).

References

Anda, R. F., Felitti, V. J., Bremner, J. D., Walker, J. D., Whitfield, C., Perry, B. D., Dube, S. R. & Giles, W. H. (2006). The enduring effects of abuse and related adverse experiences in childhood. A convergence of evidence from neurobiology and epidemiology. *European Archives of Psychiatry and Clinical Neuroscience*, 256(3), 174–186. https://doi.org/10.1007/s00406-005-0624-4.

Baquedano-López, P., Alexander, R. A. & Hernandez, S. J. (2013). Equity issues in parental and community involvement in schools: What teacher educators need to know. *Review of Educational Research*, 37, 137–149. Doi: 10.3102/0091732X12459718.

Berger, E. H., & Riojas-Cortez, M. R. (2020). *Families as partners in education: Families and schools working together* (10th ed.). Hoboken, NJ: Pearson Education.

Bethell, C., Davis, M., Gombojav, N., Stumbo, S. & Powers, K. (2017). *Issue brief: A national and across state profile on adverse childhood experiences among children and possibilities to heal and thrive.* Johns Hopkins Bloomberg School of Public Health. Retrieved from www.cahmi.org/wp-content/uploads/2018/05/aces_brief_final.pdf.

Bishop, R. S. (1990). Mirrors, windows, and sliding glass doors. Originally published in Perspectives, 1(3), ix–xi. Retrieved from https://scenicregional.org/wp-content/uploads/2017/08/Mirrors-Windows-and-Sliding-Glass-Doors.pdf.

Brandt, K. (2020). *Reflective supervision*. Bruce Perry office hours. Retrieved from https://vimeo.com/406307258.

Cooper, C. W. (2009). Performing cultural work in demographically chan-ging schools: Implications for expanding transformative leadership frameworks. *Educational Administration Quarterly, 45*(5), 649–724.

DiAngelo, R. (2016). *What does it mean to be White? Developing White racial literacy, Revised ed.,* New York, NY : Peter Lang.

Ginwright, S. (2018). *The future of healing: Shifting from trauma informed care to healing centered engagement.* Medium. Retrieved from https://medium.com/@ginwright/the-future-of-healing -shifting-from-trauma-informed-care-to-healing-centered-engagement-634f557ce69c.

Grant, K., & Ray, J. (Eds.). (2019). *Home, school, and community collabor-ation: Culturally responsive family engagement* (4th ed.). Thousand Oaks, CA: Sage.

Holochwost, S. J., DeMott, K., Buell, M., Yannetta, K. & Amsden, D. (2009) Retention of staff in the early childhood education workforce *Child & Youth Care Forum, 38*(5), 227–237. https://doi.org/10.1007/s10566-009-9078-6.

Ippolito, J. (2015). Reading interventionist research in two urban elem-entary schools through a discursive lens. *Urban Education, 26,* 1–26.

Ishimaru, A. M. (2014a). Rewriting the rules of engagement: Elaborating a model of district- community collaboration. *Harvard Educational Review, 84*(2).

Ishimaru, A. M. (2014b). When new relationships meet old narratives: The journey towards improving parent-school relations in a district-community organizing collaboration. *Teachers College Record, 116*(2).

Ishimaru, A. M. (2017). From family engagement to equitable col-laboration. *Educational Policy,* 33(4). https://doi.org/10.1177/0895904817691841.

Ishimaru, A., Lott, J., Torres, K., & O-Reilly-Diaz K. (2019). Families in the driver's seat: Catalyzing familial transformative agency for equit-able collaboration, *Teachers College Record, 121*(11), 1–39. www.tcrecord.org ID Number: 22819.

Kendi, I. X. (2019). *How to be an antiracist.* New York, NY: One World.

Mediratta, K., Shah, S. & McAlister, S. (2009). *Community organizing for stronger schools: Strategies and successes.* Cambridge, MA: Harvard Education Press.

Muhs, M. (2019). *Family engagement in early childhood settings*. St. Paul, MN: Redleaf Press.

National Academies of Sciences, Engineering, and Medicine. (2015). *Transforming the workforce for children birth through age 8: A unifying foundation*. Washington, DC.

National Association for Family, School, and Community Engagement (NAFSCE) Policy Council. (2010). *Family engagement*. Retrieved from http://nafsce.org/whowe-are/#dfe.

National Center on Parent, Family, and Community Engagement (NCPFCE). (2013). *Understanding family engagement outcomes: Research to practice series—Family connections to peers and community*. Washington, DC: U.S. Department of Health and Human Services, Administration for Children and Families, Office of Head Start, and Office of Child Care. Retrieved from https://eclkc.ohs.acf. hhs.gov/ sites/default/files/pdf/rtp-family-connections-to-peers-and-community.pdf.

National Center on Parent, Family, and Community Engagement (NCPFCE). (2014). *Building partnerships: Guide to developing relationships with families*. Washington, DC: U.S. Department of Health and Human Services, Administration for Children and Families, Office of Head Start, and Office of Child Care. Retrieved from https://eclkc.ohs.acf.hhs.gov/hslc/tta-system/family/docs/ building-partnershipsdeveloping-relationships-families.pdf.

National Research Council, Institute of Medicine. (2000). *From neurons to neighborhoods: The science of early childhood development*. Washington, DC: National Academy Press.

Nicholson, J., Perez, L. & Kurtz, J. (2019). *Trauma-informed practices for early childhood educators: Relationship-based approaches that support healing and build resilience in young children*. New York, NY: Routledge.

Olivos, E. M. (2006). *The power of parents: A critical perspective of bicultural parent involvement in public schools*. New York, NY: Peter Lang.

Padilla, C., & Thomson, D. (2021). More than one in four Latino and Black households with children are experiencing three or more hardships during COVID-19. *Child trends*. Retrieved from www. childtrends.org/publications/more-than-one-in-four-latino-and-black-households-with-children-are-experiencing-three-or-more-hardships-during-covid-19Reedy & McGrath, 2010.

Reedy, C., & McGrath, W. (2010). Can you hear me now? Staff–parent communication in child care centres. Early Child Development and Care, 180(3), 347–357. doi: 10.1080/03004430801908418.

U.S. Department of Health and Human Services, Administration for Children and Families, Office of Head Start, National Center on Parent, Family, and Community Engagement. (USDHHS) (2018). Key Indicators of High-Quality Family Engagement for Quality Rating Improvement Systems.

Warren, M. R., Hong, S., Rubin, C. H. & Uy, P. (2009). Beyond the bake sale: A community-based relational approach to parent engagement in schools. *Teachers College Record, 111*(9), 2209–2254.

Warren, M., Mapp, K. & The Community Organizing and School Reform Project. (2011). *A match on dry grass: Community organizing as a catalyst for school reform*. New York, NY: Oxford University Press.

Wells, N., Bronheim, S., Zyzanski, S. & Hoover, C. (2015). Psychometric evaluation of a consumer-developed family-centered care assessment tool. *Maternal and Child Health Journal, 19*(9), 1899–1909.

1

When We Talk About Parents and Families, Who Is Included?

Family engagement is a family-centered, strengths-based approach to establishing and maintaining relationships with families and accomplishing change together…Family engagement happens in the home, early childhood programs, and the community. It is a shared responsibility of all those who want children to succeed in school and in life. Parents and others who care for their children work together to prepare children for success. When families, communities, and early learning programs work together, young children are more successful and the entire community benefits.

(*Quality Counts California Family Engagement Toolkit,* 2019, p. 4)

When We Talk About Parents and Families, Who Is Included?

Before we can discuss trauma-responsive family engagement, we have to establish a shared understanding for what we mean when we refer to "parents" and "families." When we use these terms, we strive to acknowledge all adult caregivers who have a meaningful role in a child's life. Specifically:

♦ **Parents** refers to biological, adoptive, and step-parents as well as primary caregivers, such as grandparents, other

DOI: 10.4324/9781003127666-2

adult family members, kinship caregivers and foster or resource parents

◆ **Families** can be biological or nonbiological, chosen or circumstantial. They are connected through culture, language, tradition, shared experiences, emotional commitment, and mutual support (ECLKC, n.d., p. 1).

Traditional Approaches to Working with Parents and Families

We need to understand the difference between family involvement and family engagement. One of the dictionary definitions of involve is to "enfold or envelop," whereas one of the meanings of engagement implies engage is "to come together and interlock." Thus, involvement implies doing to; in contrast, engagement implies doing with. A school striving for family involvement often leads with its mouth—identifying projects, needs, and goals and then telling parents how they can contribute. A school striving for parent engagement, on the other hand, tends to lead with its ears—listening to what parents think, dream, and worry about. The goal of family engagement is not to serve clients but to gain partners.

(Ferlazzo, 2011, pp. 10–11)

Historically, early childhood programs have interacted with parents and families using an approach described as *parent and family involvement*. Traditional strategies for parent and family involvement include sharing information with parents about school events, offering parenting advice, organizing volunteering activities for parents (e.g., driving on field trips) and encouraging parents to reinforce the school/program's expectations and learning activities in the home (see Epstein, 1992).

Parents participate in activities, attend meetings and special events and "take advantage of opportunities at their child's early care and learning setting."

(USDHHS, 2018, p. 3)

Characteristics of Parent–Family Involvement

♦ **Based in deficit thinking.** Many parent and family involvement strategies are based in deficit thinking as they inherently seek to "fix" or "remediate" parents and incentivize changes to their behavior to better align with dominant values, norms and expectations (Baquedano-López, Alexander & Hernandez, 2013; Gutiérrez, Baquedano-López & Alvarez, 2000; Ishimaru & Takahashi, 2017).

♦ **"Doing to"**: An early childhood program using a family involvement approach, *"leads with its mouth"* (Ferlazzo, 2012). What does that mean? Topics and goals for parents' and families' education, events and activities are often *predetermined* and led/facilitated by the school or program staff or outside experts (Ferlazzo, 2012). Parents and families are told how they can contribute. This is referred to as a **school-centric approach** (Lawson, 2003) and often positions parents as passive and complacent (Baquedano-López et al., 2013) as they are rarely perceived or invited—especially nondominant[1] parents—as having the capacity or given the opportunities to influence decision-making in the early-learning program or school.

♦ **One-way communication.** Communication and requests for parent and family involvement is typically initiated by program staff and intended to go in one direction (Ferlazzo, 2011):

School/Program → → → → Parents and Families

For example: A teacher might call a family to share information about a child's behavior at preschool; an expert on early literacy might share recommended practices for book reading in the home at a parent meeting; a newsletter might offer information on a new discipline policy; an automated phone call welcomes parents to a new school year or an email is sent with requests for donations or volunteer support for a program food drive.

◆ **Focused on "what happens here."** Parent and family involvement efforts focus on their roles within the "four walls of the school" (Ferlazzo, 2012, p. 2).

Involvement Is "Necessary but Not Sufficient"

Parent and family involvement is associated with many benefits for children, families and early childhood programs. Involvement is the primary approach used in early childhood programs, schools and agencies. One way to think about involvement is a "necessary but not sufficient" approach to working with parents and families. If you have a strong involvement program at your site, continue doing what is working well and what you are proud of. And, build awareness about the limitations of this approach

Limitations of "Involvement" Approaches

It's not that family involvement is bad. Almost all the research says that any kind of increased parent interest and support of students can help. But almost all the research also says that family engagement can produce even better results—for students, for families, for schools, and for their communities.

(Ferlazzo, 2011)

As described above, a major concern of parent and family involvement approaches are the **deficit assumptions that position parents and families as "lacking and in need of support"** (see Valencia, 1991, 2011) in knowledge, skills, capacity, motivation, care, ability and promise. Schools, programs and agencies are positioned as the "experts" who can "fix" parents and their children to better conform to the school's or society's expectations (often White, Eurocentric and middle-class). Parents might be described as partners but the "partnerships" may unfortunately frame parents as problems (Baquedano-López, et al, 2013). Deficit language and assumptions are the root of cycles of oppression, prejudice, discrimination and bias (Valencia, 2011). They negatively impact "*all* parents, but the negative equity outcomes of these beliefs and practices particularly affect parents from nondominant backgrounds" (Baquedano-López et al., 2013, p. 150).

> The traditional model of parent involvement often boils down to well-intentioned efforts to "fix" individual parents so that they better conform to the school's expectations (Ishimaru et al., 2019). The term parent involvement typically suggests a view wherein parents are involved in ways defined by the school and directed towards achieving goals that parents have no part in setting. In this type of relationship, power is held by the school rather than being shared between the school and the families (Gillanders, Iruka, Bagwell, Morgan & Garcia, 2014, p. 125).

Parent and family involvement does not acknowledge **how power, race, culture, class, immigration, ability, gender and language impact the inequitable contexts that influence families' opportunities and experiences with involvement** (Baquedano-López, Alexander & Hernandez, 2013; Fine, 1993; Gutiérrez & Vossoughi, 2009; Olivos, 2006). By ignoring these factors, traditional family involvement policies and "best practices" have imagined early childhood programs, schools and agencies as neutral spaces that position everyone equally. This ignores our nation's history of institutional racism and the differential treatment of families including the types of involvement they are invited to participate in (Baquedano-López et al., 2013).

The Shift towards Family Engagement

> The shift for me after 28 years of doing this work with families is turning it over from a deficit based perspective ("they're in need or they need to learn or change something") to an asset-informed approach ("they know their child best").
>
> (Shawn Bryant, Founding Director & Chief Learning Officer at Teaching Excellence Center)

> The goal of family engagement is not to serve clients but to gain partners.
>
> (Ferlazzo, 2011, p. 2)

> The perspective of home-school partnership requires that teachers view families as a resource rather than a liability.
>
> (Gillanders, McKinney & Richie, 2012, p. 132)

Increasingly, researchers, policymakers, child and family advocates and early childhood professionals are rejecting the deficit-based assumptions underlying traditional parent education and involvement approaches and recognizing that the only way to effectively support children's learning and healthy development is to build trusting relationships with parents and families and to collaboratively engage with them in power-sharing partnerships. *Parent and family engagement* differs from a parent and family involvement approach in several ways.

Characteristics of a Parent and Family Engagement Approach

◆ **Strength-based and asset-informed: "Doing with."** In a genuine partnership, all participants teach and learn from one another and everyone is assumed to have valuable contributions to share. Aligned with this belief, all families are believed to have strengths, assets, skills and knowledge about their child's learning and development that is valuable and essential for early childhood professionals to learn about. For this reason, a family engagement approach is about *"doing with"* (Ferlazzo, 2011, p. 2).

With family engagement early childhood programs lead *with their ears*. They value and invest in relationship-building with a focus on listening to and learning from families about many things including: their beliefs, values and goals for their child's care and education; what they dream about and desire for their children's learning and development; what worries them and/or the stressors and challenges they face; how they cope and what their family's strengths, funds of knowledge (Moll, Amanti, Neff & Gonzalez, 1992), skills and forms of resilience are; the resources and forms of support they desire or need and the ways of supporting and engaging with their child and the early-learning program that are accessible and meaningful to them (Ferlazzo, 2011, p. 2).

◆ **Acknowledging a wider and range of beliefs and actions that parents and family members do to support their children.** Family engagement approaches recognize that the extraordinary diversity among parents and families of young children (ethnically/culturally, linguistically, etc.) translates into many ways of knowing, being and supporting young children. Engagement is not limited to participating in events or meetings at the school or within the four walls of the early-learning program or reproducing early-learning activities in the home. Instead, engaging in children's learning and development is recognized to be a diverse range of values, cultural routines and interactive activities especially situated within the everyday interactions within families (Auerbach, 2007; Barton et al., 2004; Fine, 1993; Galindo & Medina, 2009).

In my dissertation, I examined how parents from marginalized groups defined their own involvement in their children's education. I discovered that, sometimes, this involvement aligned with educators' expectations—like when caregivers spent time reading with children, helping with homework and volunteering. More often, however, the examples caregivers used to describe their engagement did not align with what educators frequently identify as family involvement. Parents and guardians described teaching cultural lessons and supporting social emotional learning. They engaged with their children's schooling by relocating to change school districts and navigating social services to ensure their children's needs were met. Educators must remember there are many ways for families to engage. We must recognize that all families care about their children's education and that engagement can vary based on many factors, including caregivers' cultures and beliefs, their own educational experiences, their types of employment, responsibilities to others and more. The need to broaden definitions of family involvement…is more important than ever.

(Teaching Tolerance, 2018)

◆ **Two-way communication.** Engagement involves communication that is bidirectional:

Parents and Families ← → Early Childhood Program

Efforts are made to communicate in ways that are accessible, culturally responsive and translated into home languages. Additionally, multiple pathways are provided for families to communicate and engage their voices, e.g., during home visits, phone calls/texts, surveys, parent advocacy groups, parent membership on boards, with parent assigned advocates and more. Communication flows back and forth.

◆ **Power-sharing that supports parent and family voice and agency.** Parent/family education, events and activities are co-designed and families have leadership roles and influence in shaping the agendas, topics, formats and goals to be responsive to their interests and needs. Parents and family members also have leadership roles to organize and facilitate family-centered events and experiences. Programs may have coordinators that work as liaisons between the parent communities and the early childhood programs.

Parents and families are believed to have valuable insights about how to improve/transform early childhood programs, schools and services to be more equitable and responsive to the needs of children and families, especially those farthest from opportunity and resources (Ishimaru et al., 2019). Parents and families have opportunities for agency to intervene and advocate on behalf of their children and to contribute to changes that disrupt inequitable policies and practices and remove barriers to access and opportunities for their children's healthy development and learning (Baquedano-López, et al., 2013).

◆ **A willingness to go beyond families' interests and concerns "within the four walls of the program" to acknowledge the pressing issues within the community where the program is located and where parents and families live.** Just as parent involvement tends to focus solely on concerns and improving what goes on within the four walls of the early-learning program, family engagement invites families to bring in the larger issues they are facing in their lives when thinking about programming and/or connecting families to community resources. For example, Laura Rivas, Family Engagement Specialist understands that the prevalence of housing instability for families in her school is an important focus for her school's family engagement efforts.

Sometimes we approach families as if we don't see them as part of the larger community. Maybe we don't feel we have the capacity to go into the community or to understand. Where my school is located, how can I not look at the reality of gentrification and how that's impacting the children and families in our community? The housing crisis is huge here. There are so many other things too, but homelessness is a huge issue. We have children probably in every other classroom in our schools that have at one point been homeless. And how often did teachers talk about homelessness in the classroom? I think it's very rare. We talk about other things that children may or may not be able to relate to. But the wealth gap that exists in our city, it's one of the biggest in the nation. And yet it's really hard to find books and other resources that address class differences for children but children in our schools deal with these things all the time. And in our classrooms there are all these little ways that these realities impact children, but we're not talking about it

(Laura Rivas, Family Engagement Specialist,
Berkeley Unified School District)

Power-Sharing That Supports Parent and Family Voice and Agency

"The Parents began by Developing the Menu"—Mayra Cruz, faculty De Anza College and former Executive Director of Community Family Services, Inc.

Mayra Cruz was a program administrator at Community Family Services, Inc., an early childhood and family services organization, and was responsible for planning and supervising the use of federal and state funds to support the agency. She explains how her agency worked in power-sharing partnership with parents and centered their voices and agency in decision-making about the program policies and practices:

One of the aspects about family support that I learned early on was how we could engage our parents and families to help us determine the needs, the wishes and the dreams that collectively we wanted to address as an organization. Our parents began by gathering with us. We had chart paper all over the room, and then there were some inquiry questions like, "what is it that we need to do to support your wellbeing and your development as families?" And so we created what we all called "the menu." The parents began by developing this menu and it became the tool for our organization to develop current and future programs and services. But then what happened after that was even better. After the development of "the menu," the families had the power and choice to decide which ways they wanted to be involved and to impact the organization, a parent advisory committee was formed; we called it the Parent Council, and the Parent Council was powerful. They were the ones who evaluated their goals and the menu annually and they helped us evaluate the whole program, and then determine the directions that we needed to go. Families were able to choose the types and levels of involvement across a spectrum that they designed that provided opportunities for parents to get involved in the way that they wanted to be involved. Our approach was based on honoring the parents' strengths and assets. We never said, "we can't." We worked in collaboration with families to be about dreaming and creating the possibilities with them.

Reflection/Discussion Question

◆ In what ways do you provide opportunities for families to create their own menu? To have a voice and input to inform decisions the program will make that will impact them?

"Having Humility is So Important"—Laura Rivas, Family Engagement Specialist, Berkeley Unified School District

Laura Rivas, Family Engagement Specialist, in a large urban school district describes how small acts of listening, humility and taking a stance of "there is space for both my knowledge and the families' knowledge in this room" is central to family engagement:

> Too often as a school staff, we come with an agenda and we deeply believe that our agenda is the best thing for the child, we believe we know what's best for a child or what's best for a family. And deep down, we believe that we know better than they do. Even me, as a Latina from a working-class background, I went to college, I had access to a master's degree education which gave me access to certain levels of institutional knowledge that could impact me in thinking that now, I know better. I have the lived experience of a working-class upbringing and the institutional knowledge so I might think, "I know better." But **having humility is so important**. Yes, I may have a multifaceted approach informed by my lived experiences *and* there is value in approaching a community with humility. Typically school staff, early educators, we weren't raised in the community that we're working with.

Laura understands the difference between family involvement (doing to) and family engagement (doing with) and conveys this beautifully in her own words. She embodies family engagement as she is prioritizing listening to families' thoughts, feelings, ideas, worries and opinions instead of just listening to her own ideas and/or agenda of what she thinks is best for a family. She extends an invitation for a two-way partnership, a mutual conversation where they partner together to come up with solutions. This "humility" she talks about is simply taking the stance, "I don't know everything, families are experts too and we need to listen with our hearts, not just with our ears."

Although both parent/family involvement and parent/family engagement approaches are beneficial, the empirical evidence is almost universal in describing family engagement as more effective and associated with a wider range of positive outcomes for children, families, programs and schools, and communities (Baquedano-López, Alexander & Hernandez, 2013; Ferlazzo & Hammond, 2009). Most early childhood programs will strive to have aspects of parent and family involvement *and* parent and family engagement. Review the differences in the table below.

Key characteristics and distinctions
(Ferlazzo, 2012)

Parent or family INVOLVEMENT	*Parent or family ENGAGEMENT*
Involvement implies "Doing to" Definition: "to enfold or envelope."	Engagement implies "Doing with" Definition: "to come together and interlock."
A school striving for family involvement often **leads with its mouth**—identifying projects, needs and goals and then telling parents how they can contribute.	Interactive process of relationship-building built on listening.
Invitations for parent involvement often come through **one-way** forms of communication—exchange of information about the child, offering advice or recommending resources to address challenges, notes home, automated phone calls, or requests for assistance for a particular project. Often **initiated by educators/programs**.	A school focused on family engagement will **lead with their ears**, listening to parents' and family members' ideas and learn about their hopes, dreams and worries for their children as well as what they believe works best for their child.
Parents **participate in activities, attend meetings and special events** and take advantage of opportunities at their child's early care and learning setting.	Engagement strives to utilize **two-way** conversation, through efforts like making home visits and phone calls that are not limited to concerns and problems.
Topics and goals for parent/family nights and events are often **pre-determined** by the school and led and taught by school staff or outside experts.	Communication is mutual, respectful, and **responsive to a family's language and culture**.
	We **partner with families** to share responsibility for the care and learning of children.
	Curricula for parent/family nights and events are responsive to the topics that families are interested in learning about. **Parents/family members take a leadership role** in planning and facilitating meetings and feel a sense of ownership in shaping the agendas and goals. Often, Parent Coordinators act as liaisons between the parent communities and the school or program.

Key characteristics and distinctions
(Ferlazzo, 2012)

Parent or family INVOLVEMENT	Parent or family ENGAGEMENT
Focus is upon improving what goes on **within the four walls of the school.**	School/program participating as an institution **within the larger community** (e.g., collaborates with local religious congregations, businesses, neighborhood groups and non-profit agencies to tackle community challenges (e.g., violence, housing, food insecurity etc.)).

Reflection/Discussion Questions

♦ In reviewing the left column in the chart above, are there examples of how you and/or your program practice **Family Involvement**?

♦ In reviewing the right column in the chart above, are there examples of how you and/or your program practice **Family Engagement**?

Note

1 Non-dominant parents: "Communities who have traditionally been marginalized or underserved by dominant institutions, practices and power relations, such as low-income, immigrant/refugee, and other communities of color" (Gutiérrez, 2006; Ishimaru, Lott, Torres & O-Reilly-Diaz, 2019).

References

Auerbach, S. (2007). From moral supporters to struggling advocates: Reconceptualizing parent roles in education through the experience of working-class families of color. *Urban Education, 42,* 250–283. doi:10.1177/0042085907300433.

Baquedano-López, P., Alexander, R. A. & Hernandez, S. J. (2013). Equity issues in parental and community involvement in schools: What teacher educators need to know. *Review of Educational Research, 37*, 137–149. doi: 10.3102/0091732X12459718.

Barton, A. C., Drake, C., Perez, J. G., St. Louis, K. & George, M. (2004). Ecologies of parental engagement in urban education. *Educational Researcher, 33*, 3–12. doi:10.3102/ 0013189X033004003.

Early Childhood Learning and Knowledge Center (ECLKC). (nd). *Parent involvement and family engagement. For early childhood professionals.* Office of Head Start, Administration of Children and Families. https://eclkc.ohs.acf.hhs.gov/sites/default/files/pdf/parent-involvement-family-engagement-forprofessionals.pdf.

Epstein, J. L. (1992). School and family partnerships. In M. Alkin (Ed.), *Encyclopedia of educational research* (pp. 1139–1151). New York, NY: Macmillan.

Ferlazzo, L. (2011). Involvement or engagement? *Educational Leadership: Schools, Families, Communities, 68*(8), 10–14.

Ferlazzo, L. (2012). Response: The difference between parent "involvement" and parent "engagement." *Education Week Teacher.* https://blogs.edweek.org/teachers/classroom_qa_with_larry_ferlazzo/2012/03/response_the_difference_between_parent_involvement_parent_engagement.html.

Ferlazzo, L., & Hammond, L. A. (2009). *Building parent engagement in schools.* Santa Barbara, CA: Linworth.

Fine, M. 1993. [Ap]parent involvement: Reflections on parents, power, and urban public schools. *Teachers College Record, 94*, 4, 682–708.

Galindo, R., & Medina, C. (2009). Cultural appropriation, performance, and agency in Mexicana parent involvement. *Journal of Latinos in Education, 8*, 312–331. doi:10.1080/15348430902973450.

Gillanders, C., Iruka, I., Bagwell, C., Morgan, J. & Garcia, S. (2014). Home and school partnerships: Raising children together. In S. Ritchie & L. Gutmann (Eds.), *First school: Transforming PreK-3rd grade for African American, Latino, and low-income children* (pp. 125–148). New York, NY: Teachers College Press.

Gillanders, C., McKinney, M. & Ritchie, S. (2012). What type of school would you like for your children? Exploring minority mothers' beliefs to promote home-school partnerships. *Early Childhood Education Journal, 40*(5), 285–94.

Gutiérrez, K., Baquedano-López, P. & Alvarez, H. (2000). The crisis in Latino education: The norming of America. In C. Tejeda, C. Martínez, & Z.

Leonardo (Eds.), *Charting new terrains in Chicano(a) and Latina(o) education* (pp. 213–232). Cresskill, NJ: Hampton Press.

Gutierrez, K. D., & Vossoughi, S. (2009). Lifting off the ground to return anew: Mediated praxis, transformative learning, and social design experiments. *Journal of Teacher Education, 61*(1–2), 100–117.

Ishimaru, A., Lott, J., Torres, K. & O-Reilly-Diaz, K. (2019). Families in the driver's seat: Catalyzing familial transformative agency for equitable collaboration. *Teachers College Record, 121*(11), 1–39. www.tcrecord.org ID Number: 22819.

Ishimaru, A. M., & Takahashi, S. (2017). Disrupting racialized institutiona scripts: Towards parent-teacher transformative agency for educational justice. *Peabody Journal of Education*. Retrieved from http:/. dx.doi.org/10.1080/0161956X.2017.1324660.

Lawson, M. A. (2003). School-family relationships in context: Parent and teacher perceptions of parent involvement. *Urban Education, 3ε*, 77–133.

Moll, L. C., Amanti, C., Neff, D. & Gonzalez, N. (1992). Funds of knowledge for teaching: Using a qualitative approach to connect homes and classrooms. *Theory Into Practice, 31*(2), 132–141.

Olivos, E. M. (2006). *The power of parents: A critical perspective of bicultural parent involvement in public schools*. New York, NY: Peter Lang.

Quality Counts California (2019). *Family engagement resource guide: Family engagement toolkit*. First 5 California. Retrieved from https://qualitycountsca.net/child-care-providers/family-engagement/family-engagement-toolkit/.

Teaching Tolerance (2018). *Critical practices for anti-bias education*. Retrieved from www.tolerance.org/magazine/publications/critical-practices-for-antibias-education.

U.S. Department of Health and Human Services, Administration for Children and Families, Office of Head Start, National Center on Parent, Family, and Community Engagement. (USDHHS) (2018). Key Indicators of High-Quality Family Engagement for Quality Rating Improvement Systems.https://childcareta.acf.hhs.gov/sites/default/files/public/indicators-final-508.pdf.

Valencia, R. (1991). *Chicano school failure and success: Research and policy agendas for the 1990s*. New York, NY: Falmer.

Valencia, R. (2011). *Chicano school failure and success: Past, present, and future* (3rd ed.). London: Routledge.

2

Understanding State Dependent Functioning: The Importance of Maintaining Regulation in Trauma-Responsive Environments

State Dependent Functioning

Trauma-responsive practice is guided by an understanding of the neurobiology of stress and trauma or what Bruce Perry (2020a) describes as **state dependent functioning**. State dependent functioning means:

♦ **Our internal state is always changing along an arousal continuum** (Perry, 2020a). Our state of emotions/stress may move up and down the arousal continuum throughout the day. As we rise up the continuum, our stress response system becomes more activated, and we move closer to hyperarousal (fight, flight) or hypoarousal (freeze). As we move down the continuum our stress response system becomes less activated and we move closer to calm, thinking more clearly and accessing the part of our brain that can solve problems for the greater good.

DOI: 10.4324/9781003127666-3

◆ **Our perceptions of threat and fear are especially impactful in shifting our internal states.** Our brains are continually receiving input from multiple sensory domains (e.g., what we hear, see, smell, taste, touch, feel and our past experiences) to monitor our internal state and the external environment to scan for safety or danger.

Our brain functioning is state dependent. The dynamic activity of all networks in the brain shifts in response to internal and external stimuli. Therefore, the "capability" of a person in any given moment is fluid; your cognitive, emotional, social, motor and regulatory capabilities shift with your internal state. Fear mobilizes some networks and capabilities while shutting down others.

(Perry, 2020a)

◆ **The more distressed and fearful we are, the more we move up the arousal continuum** shifting away from a calm state into an alert state, then alarm, then fear followed by being in a state of terror which is the most stressed state we can be in.

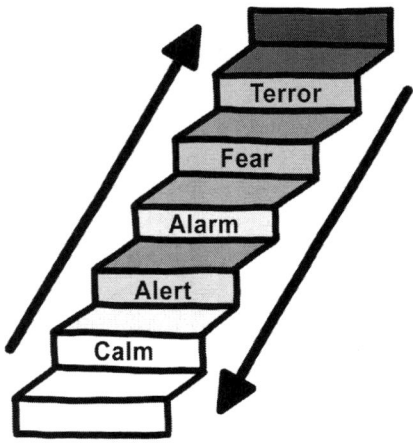

FIGURE 2.1
Arousal continuum
Source: Alice Blecker

We know from decades of research that several characteristics amplify a stress response for individuals and for groups reducing peoples' feelings of safety and moving them farther up the arousal continuum (calmness → alarm, fear and terror). These characteristics include:

- **Novelty**. Events or experiences that are new, unfamiliar or that create uncertainty can lead our brains to perceive danger and can activate our stress response system
- **Unpredictability.** Events or experiences we go through where there is a significant level of uncertainty and a constant sense of change, can elevate our stress
- **Lack of personal agency and control.** When people do not perceive they have a sense of agency and control, feelings of fear, anxiety and hypervigilance increase which activates our stress response and moves us up the arousal continuum

> In the same way that children exhibit state dependent functioning, so do adults, families, programs, organizations, schools, communities, businesses, governments and countries.
>
> (Perry, 2020a)

Our brainstem and limbic brain are continually receiving input from multiple sensory systems (e.g., what we hear, see, smell, taste, feel and/or our past experiences etc.) and monitoring our internal state and the external environment to determine if we are safe or in danger.

When the Cortex Is "Open" for Business
When adults perceive that they are safe and not threatened in any way, as Bruce Perry describes, "their cortex is open for business."

The Pre-Frontal Cortex or Neo-Cortex (Executive or Thinking Brain)

Mammals and reptiles do not have a neo-cortex. Only humans have a neo-cortex allowing us to have more advanced processing capabilities. The neo-cortex is considered the **"Boss or Chief Executive Officer"** of the brain.

When adults are calm and regulated, have their basic needs met (e.g., enough food and water, neither hot or cold), do not have excessive demands on their attention, are in a familiar environment and/or with people they trust and they have a felt sense of belonging and safety, they can engage the full range of their cognitive reasoning and capabilities. That is, their "cortex is open for business." This means they are capable of:

- ◆ Engaging in reflection
- ◆ Identifying how they feel and how intense their emotions are
- ◆ Thinking abstractly
- ◆ Creating and inventing
- ◆ Learning new information

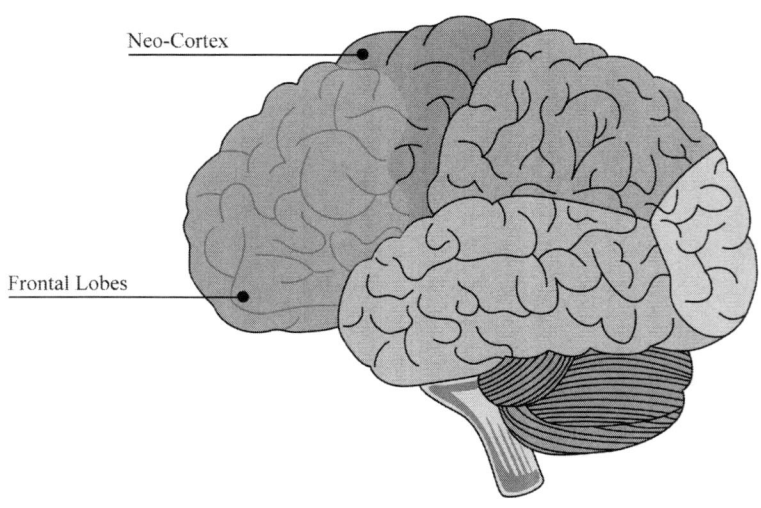

FIGURE 2.2
Neo-cortex
Source: Courtney Vickery

- Relating to time in complex ways (considering the past and dreaming into the future)
- Making thoughtful decisions after considering different ideas and solutions
- Examining different perspectives (other than one's own)
- Problem-posing and problem-solving
- Using strategies to self-regulate emotions and behavior
- Aligning their beliefs and behaviors with expressed values, an organizational mission and/or an understanding of a greater good
- Thinking logically and keeping the big picture in mind while mapping out the steps to achieve a goal
- Considering the potential or actual consequences of one's beliefs, decisions and/or behaviors
- Sustaining their focal attention
- Having and expressing empathy

When the Amygdala (Built-In Alarm or Smoke Detector) Is Set Off and the Brain Detects Danger

If our brain detects any information that suggests a potential threat (**internally**: e.g., adults are hungry, thirsty, cold or emotionally triggered; **externally**: e.g., they are in an unfamiliar environment with people they don't know or trust or they feel unsafe), it will automatically and subconsciously activate the amygdala which sends a survival response and stress chemicals that engage the brainstem and limbic brain and other systems throughout the brain and body to mobilize a fight, flight or freeze survival reaction.

The Brainstem (Primitive Brain)

The brainstem is responsible for the FLIGHT, FIGHT and FREEZE response humans have when they perceive danger. This part of the brain waits for the amygdala "**alarm center**" or "**smoke detector**" to send signals to our lower brain/brainstem that we are in danger which sets off a range of physiological responses: increase in body temperature, dilation of our pupils, rapid breathing and others. Our brain and body are mobilizing to

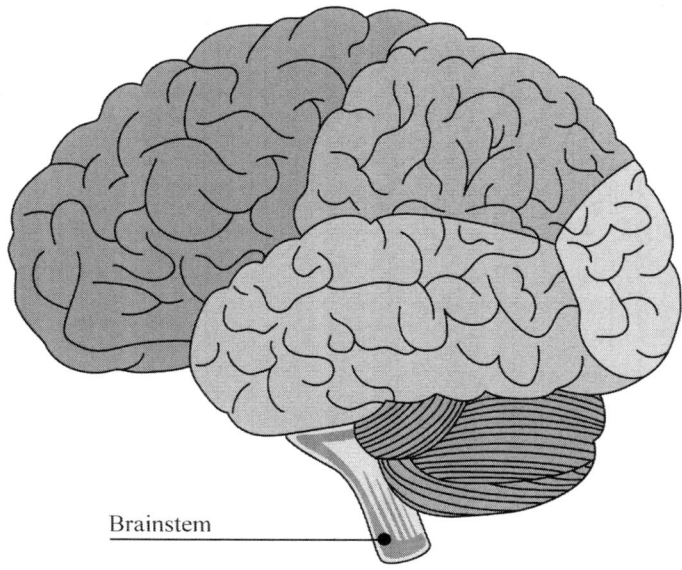

FIGURE 2.3
Brainstem
Source: Courtney Vickery

protect us from real (natural disaster, car swerves into our lane)
or perceived (uncertainty, stress, trauma reminders) danger.

The Limbic Brain (Emotional and Relational Brain)

We share this part of our brain with mammals. It generates
our feelings, the emotional intensity of feelings and our desire
for attachment, significance, and belonging. The limbic brain
supports our ability to feel a range of emotions. When we have
too much stress, our emotions can rise up and may activate the
amygdala (alarm center) and set off our lower brain to set off
a fight, flight or freeze stress response. Additionally, when we
feel isolated, disconnected, not seen or when we don't feel we
belong, these are also triggers that set off the alarm center in our
brain and start a cascade of chemicals waking up our lower brain
to protect us from real or perceived dangers by fighting, running
away or becoming immobile.

The Limbic Brain

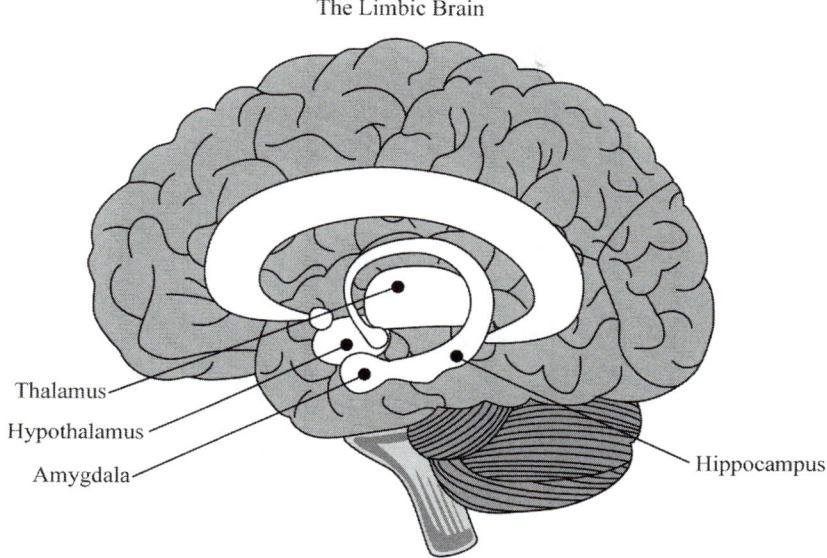

Thalamus

Hypothalamus

Amygdala

Hippocampus

FIGURE 2.4
Limbic
Source: Courtney Vickery

What Happens to Adults' Functioning as Their State Shifts and They Move Up the Arousal Continuum?

When our brains detect a threat, because of state dependent functioning, our core regulatory networks will set off a cascade of changes in how we think, what we feel and the way we behave (Perry, 2020a). Certain systems are "turned on" in our brains and bodies while others are "turned off" or less accessible and what is critical for trauma-responsive early childhood staff to understand: *the greater a person's brain and body perceives threat, the less access they will have to their cortex.* When we are under stress, the thinking parts of our brains are less functional as faster more primitive survival systems take over. There are several consequences for adults' functioning. **When the cortex is "closed for business" and less accessible/functional, adults will be more:**

◆ Reactive, emotional, anxious and activated. Reactivity, highly emotional and worried states are common characteristics of people when they are distressed and show signs of state dependent regression (moving up the arousal continuum). This might look like:

- A teacher who raises her voice with children, calls in sick frequently, shuts down emotionally and/or who is on edge and short tempered
- A parent who at drop off and pick up is always on the phone, unresponsive to communication such as emails or phone messages, becomes reactive to a comment, complains about teachers or the program, becomes critical or yells at their children frequently

The further that you escalate up the arousal continuum, the more you have what we call **state dependent regression.** You act less and less and less like an adult and more and more and more like a child and at some point you regress and get to the point where you're completely self-referential…you just care about your comfort. You want your needs met, and you want them met now… you are hard to reason with, you're emotional and reactive in the way you do things…the more you get threatened, the less access you have your cortex, and the more you basically functionally regress.

(Perry, 2020a)

◆ **Externally focused and vigilant.** Scanning for danger is a characteristic of adults who are stressed and in a state of hypervigilance. Increased sensitivity or reactivity to sound, light and touch is common. Also misreading the intentions of others during interactions or when reading and responding to written communication. This might look like:

- A site supervisor who fires off an accusatory email falsely attributing a motive to someone they super-vise before seeking to understand what happened, misinterpreting an employee's comment as an intentional attack on them, assuming an employee calls in sick because they didn't want to meet the deadline for an assignment (when they are sick), or constantly micro-managing everything the people they supervise are doing and saying.

- A parent who jumps with a startle reaction when a family engagement specialist unexpectedly approaches them from behind to chat and reacts by saying, "why are you looking at me like that?" or misinterprets a question about how their son is doing at home by saying, "Are you trying so say I am a bad parent?"

◆ **Emotionally and physically exhausted**. Having a stress response system that is continually activated and scanning the environment for danger takes a toll emotionally, physically, socially, mentally and spiritually. And this translates into less responsiveness and less ability to focus. The longer this hypervigilant state lasts, the more adults will see themselves or those around them through a negative lens and their ability to engage, participate, and to sustain attention will be significantly reduced. This might look like:

- A parent who avoids interactions, calls and/or is not responsive when you reach out with a question, concern or a reminder about paperwork deadlines.
- A caregiver who cannot console a crying baby and blames the parents for spoiling them too much by constantly holding them. Or who struggles to complete her parent newsletters or to call home to check in with families because she is too exhausted.

◆ **Less capable of being creative, inventive and reflective**. When stressed, adults may not be capable of hearing or receiving new information and they will likely struggle to engage in reflection, problem-solving, thoughtful analysis of an issue or thinking creatively and "out of the box" in planning or coming up with plans and solutions. This might look like:

- During a parent meeting, the caregiver is shut down, unable to think through solutions or to generate next steps when asked what might support a child in her class who is experiencing anxiety at naptime.

- A director leading a staff meeting wanting to brainstorm ideas for a new family engagement program. No one in the meeting is sharing input or ideas. The one person who does speak up says, "whatever you think is best we will go with."

◆ **Focused on the current moment**. Stress, especially at the high end of the arousal continuum (alarm → fear → terror), impacts adults' ability to focus. As a result, meeting, planning and engaging in activities that require people to reflect on the past or think into the future are more difficult when people are distressed. This might look like:

- A family who is provided a list of resources they requested (food, housing, clothing) never takes the next steps to call the numbers they were provided to access the resources.
- Families who have difficulty completing required paperwork, tasks or program requirements for enrollment for the new year.

◆ **Less capable of thinking through the outcomes or consequences of their behavior and the potential impact to themselves, others and the group.** When adults are stressed, decisions can become impulsive, irrational or overly focused on meeting immediate needs instead of considering what is the best long-term outcome and/or for the greater good. Reflection on the potential impact of the choices being made is less likely to take place. This might look like:

- A parent that goes from 0–100 emotionally by lashing out with words toward a family childcare provider saying, "Maybe you are not a good caregiver because you are young and don't have your own kids."
- A family member who threatens a teacher or site supervisor with removal of their child if they don't get their way.

- A family approaches their child's speech therapist with a request for more speech therapy and the speech therapist says, "maybe if you worked more with your child at home that would help."

◆ **Making lower quality decisions.** The quality of adults' decision-making begins to deteriorate—they experience decision fatigue (Perry, 2020b)—when their brains detect stress (e.g., basic needs not being met, high stress, uncertainty and a lack of control). As an adult becomes stressed, dysregulated and/or in a state of alarm, their decisions and ability to problem-solve are compromised. They are not as thoughtful or future-oriented (they are focused on survival) and they are more likely to react based on their biases and prejudices and/or to be simplistic in their thinking and solutions (e.g., less likely to focus on nuance, context or specific circumstances). Decision fatigue is most impactful when adults have to make lots of decisions in a row. This might look like:

  - A team is meeting to discuss the results of a screening assessment completed with a young toddler and her family to determine what services she qualifies for. They wait until right before lunch when everyone in the room is tired and hungry to make the most important decisions. Despite the father's request for speech therapy twice a week, everyone is tired and hungry and motivated to end the meeting quickly. So a quick decision is made to take a "wait and see" approach and not to approve the father's request at this time. The family leaves anxious and upset that the decision was made quickly and without careful consideration. They worry that their child's development may suffer as a result.

  - A community is impacted by a Category 5 hurricane. Following this catastrophic event, early childhood programs mobilized quickly. Meeting after meeting is convened to create handouts and resources for parents on how to support their children, lists of community resources are generated and emergency crisis units are mobilized to support families who lost their homes. Staff work around the clock with very little sleep. The lack of sleep, sense of urgency and staff being on high alert take a toll and only later everyone realizes that they forgot to ask families what *they* needed/wanted.

◆ **Showing a range of behavioral changes.** When stressed, adults will show a range of behaviors. Some may become hypervigilant and constantly scan the environment for information to determine if they are safe. This may include observing what other people are doing, their tone, facial expressions, behaviors or what they are saying. In this hypervigilant state, there may be misinterpretations of those verbal and nonverbal clues causing them to become defiant and aggressive or to respond with compliance, a dissociative response, that supports coping in the face of a perceived threat (Perry, 2020a). This might look like:

- A principal welcomes a grandparent who arrives at preschool for drop off saying, "good morning and how are you doing today?" The grandparent looks at her with a blank stare and walks right past the principal.
- During a developmental playgroup, the facilitator notices one of the mothers is constantly looking around the room and at her phone instead of playing with her young toddler.
- A kindergarten teacher hands a friendly reminder to the parent of one of the children in her class at pick up time. The note requests that the parent return the required emergency and immunization forms no later than the following day. The parent rips up the note and throws it in the trash on the way out.

◆ **Resistant to new conversations, changes, recommendations, feedback and suggestions.** The more threatened and unsafe adults feel, the more likely they are to be resistant to reflective conversations, change, feedback, recommendations or suggestions. For people to feel safe, their brains and bodies need to reduce the factors that increase the stress response: novelty, unpredictability and lack of agency and control. Therefore, some people will prefer to remain in a difficult situation more than changing it simply because it feels safer, is familiar, more predictable and continuing with the ways things have been done, leaves them feeling a greater sense of agency and control. This might look like:

- When a teacher suggests a meeting to discuss some emerging concerns and a parent reacts by saying "I don't have any time and that is your job to figure out."
- A family engagement specialist says to a parent, "would you like to sign up for our new parenting class we are offering for free to all families?" The parent reacts with, "are you trying to tell me I am not a good parent?"

Stress is Contagious. So is Calmness

Human beings are relational, and therefore, we absorb the emotions or internal state of those around us. Our capacity to instinctively and immediately understand what another is feeling or experiencing is due to our **mirror neurons**. In this way, the mirror neuron system is the neurological foundation that supports humans' ability to empathize, socialize, and communicate our emotions to others. Mirror neurons are activated when an individual observes someone else taking an action (e.g., walking toward them, gesturing that they need help) or when they observe someone experiencing an emotion (e.g., fear, anger, happiness, surprise) as they help us perceive other peoples' intentions (Acharya & Shukla, 2012; Conkbayir, 2017). **One person's emotional state is "mirrored" by the neuronal system of another** as the mirror system of one person alters their emotional and physical state to match the emotional and physical state of the person they are interacting with. An example of this is when we see someone crying and feel sad knowing that they are hurting, or we sense someone is stressed and this creates our own feeling of internal distress. This process of taking-in another's emotional state happens at a subconscious level, which means we are neither aware of this process nor in control of it (Nicholson, Kurtz & Perez, 2019, p. 41).

Drew Giles, Director of Educator Programs, Franklin-McKinley School District at Educare, Silicon Valley describes how he reinforces with his staff the power of using mirror neurons to calm and regulate adults in the context of daily interactions:

> I talk to my staff about being a mirror. I am basically saying when someone comes at you with a lot of escalated energy, we don't want to absorb that energy, but instead, if we stay calm, they will then begin to absorb that calm. In this way, we can lead them to regulation rather than dysregulation.

> **When interacting with an adult or child whose stress response system has been activated, we have a choice: We can follow them down into further dysregulation or remain calm and guide them back to regulation.** Viktor Frankl says, "In between a triggering event and your reaction is a pause. In that pause we have the power to choose." We can cultivate a brief pause so we can choose how we want to respond instead of unconsciously becoming reactive. In our power to choose, we can choose to act in ways that lead others to a state of regulation. Also, when others are dysregulated or reactive, we can choose to not follow or mirror their state by matching their heightened emotions but instead, to provide co-regulation to soothe their emotional distress. It is important for early childhood professionals to demonstrate a willingness to assist families when their stress response systems are triggered. By staying with the parent or family and communicating messages of calm, empathy, care, and safety, we can support a parent to calm their stress systems.

In essence, we can use our state of regulation/calm to guide a distressed parent back to regulation. It is emotionally attuned interpersonal interactions with a reliable and trusted person that co-regulates their arousal levels (alarm, fear or terror → calm) and generates a feeling of safety (Porges, 2011).

Drew shares that remaining calm externally in their interactions with parents and families does not mean that they won't be managing a range of feelings and sensations inside their bodies. He works proactively with his staff to practice and be prepared for emotional emergencies. Just like we have fire, earthquake or hurricane drills, we also need to prepare for unexpected emotional emergencies. So, in meetings, he leads his staff through practice scenarios, "What would you do if?..." They brainstorm strategies they can use to stay calm in the present moment with a parent or family member who may be showing signs of stress. They know that if they use strategies to remain calm, that they can help their families feel safe and re-regulate them through their calm presence.

◢ Lifeline: Learning the Pathways to Regulation

To provide trauma-responsive engagement with families, adults need to be regulated to access their cortex. It is critical that early childhood professionals learn how to use various strategies to reduce their stress and calm their stress response systems when activated. *The key to trauma-responsive, attuned, equitable and high-quality practice with families is regulation.*

What Is the Most Effective and Powerful Pathway to Regulation?
Relational Regulation used with one or more of the following forms of regulation:

- ◆ Top-down regulation
- ◆ Bottom-up regulation
- ◆ Intentional disconnection regulation

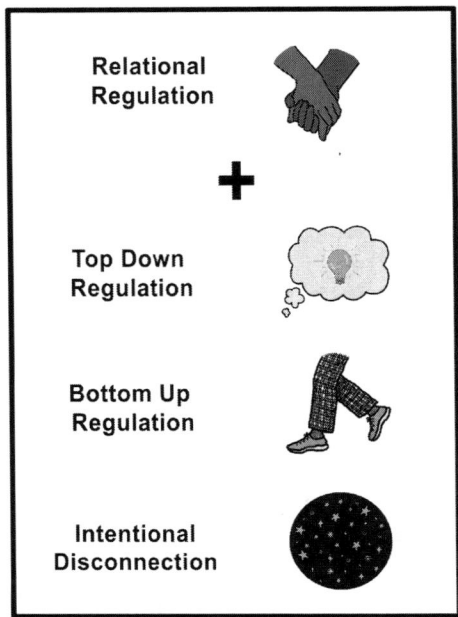

FIGURE 2.5
Relational pathways
Source: Alice Blecker

The Foundation: Relational Regulation

Relational regulation is the most powerful way to buffer stress. Families feel safest when they are with others who provide them with a sense of belonging and with whom they experience mutual feelings of care and respect. This is due to our relational neurobiology or the ways in which our brains are wired for connection. When we are in the presence of others we care for, love and respect, we can tolerate more stress and adversity and we are also more likely to have opportunities to build resilience and heal from the impact of adversity and trauma. And the reverse is also true, when families are in environments that lack a value for and focus on caring relationships, they are more vulnerable to the negative impacts of stressors and less likely to build resilience and heal from trauma.

As Perry (2020c) states, the most powerful and effective approaches to regulating our emotions and behavior happen when adults are in the presence of others they trust and feel safe with (relational regulation) and use one or more of the following strategies:

Top-Down Approaches: "Using Your Cortex (Thoughts) to Regulate and Calm"

One way to regulate and reduce stress is a "top-down" approach. This is using your cortex to help calm your stress response system by thinking or telling yourself that you are safe, that you are OK, you can handle a stressor, you may have a perceived sense of being in danger, but you are *really* safe. Top-down strategies use the intellectual parts of our brains, our thinking/reasoning, to help us calm our stress related emotions and behaviors. Top-down strategies are effective in some situations, however, they require use of the cortex. Once someone is already dysregulated and their lower brainstem is activating a survival response, it is extremely difficult to use top-down regulation strategies as the cortex can drop to as low as 10% of its efficiency when we are high on the arousal continuum (Perry, 2020c). This is why, although quite popular, top-down strategies are the least effi-cient pathway to regulation. Examples of top-down regulation strategies include:

- ◆ Thinking of grounders that can help you calm your activated stress (people, places, objects, activities associated with safety, belonging and calm)
- ◆ Mapping out different solutions to a problem or looking at all sides of a situation
- ◆ Repeating self-talk, mantras, a prayer or an inspirational saying ("I got this!" or "This too shall pass")
- ◆ Cognitive Behavioral Therapy (addressing distorted thinking patterns; changing "This is the end of the world" to "This is just a moment in time. I can get through this.")
- ◆ Journaling
- ◆ Talking about how you feel (counseling, coach, trusted confidante, mentor)

"See the Person behind the Behavior": Using a Top-Down Strategy to Regulate

A parent approached Teacher Brian with some intense emotions and pointed comments, "You folks don't seem to have experience here with children. You all seem so young and likely don't have children of your own. My child is being bullied by other kids and I am ready to report this place for neglect for letting my child get hurt!" Brian felt his heart racing, his thoughts move to "what is wrong with you" and on the tip of his tongue were comments if said aloud he knew he would regret. In the moment, he said briefly to himself, **"see the person behind the behavior"** (self-talk) and "what is this family trying to communicate that they feel or need?" (looking at all sides of the problem). Using this thought, Teacher Brian was able to calm himself and access another way to respond that was more professional and healthier. This top-down strategy disrupted his reactionary pattern and created space for a more trauma-responsive approach using his cortex. After grounding himself, he said to the parent, "I care how you feel. I want to hear more. Might we go to a private place to talk or if you prefer, schedule a time where I can be fully present to listen to how you feel and together we can find a solution?"

At the beginning of the meeting to talk about the parent's concerns, the parent entered without responding. He was greeted by Brian and said "no" to all offers of a refreshment or drink. The parent's shoulders looked tense, he looked down at the ground, had minimal and averted eye contact and his arms were crossed. Brian asked the parent if they could start by making a list of the strengths of his child (top-down strategy: looking at all sides of the problem) and then all the concerns in another column. After this activity, the parent seemed to make a humorous comment, smile, his shoulders looked more relaxed and he was more verbal and engaged in the conversation. This activity helped ground both parties by allowing the executive (thinking brain) to be accessed by writing a list a of all the issues and the strengths. This top-down strategy helped create a pathway to the executive brain so that they could start off with a more regulated and integrated approach to looking at the problem with one another.

Reflection/Discussion Questions

◆ Have you used a top-down approach to calm your activated stress response system? Can you list an example of how you used that strategy for yourself so that you could access and integrate all parts of your brain?

◆ Have you used a top-down strategy with a family you have worked with to calm their activated stress response system?

Bottom-Up Approaches: "Using Patterned Repetitive Somatosensory Activities to Regulate and Calm"

Bottom-up approaches are the fastest and most effective and direct way of regulating stress for children and adults (Perry, 2020c). Bottom-up approaches directly reach the core neural networks in the lower brain responsible for regulation. Repetitive *somato* (movement) *sensory* (sight/sound/touch etc.) activities engage these core regulatory networks and help people calm their stress and regulate their brains and bodies. Examples of bottom-up regulation strategies include:

◆ Rocking back and forth (in a rocking chair or just in place)
◆ Walking or running
◆ Swimming, riding a bike
◆ Jumping (e.g., in place or on a trampoline)
◆ Petting a dog or other pets/animals
◆ Listening to music, dancing, singing or chanting
◆ Humming
◆ Coloring, using fidget toys
◆ Deep breathing exercises

- ◆ Stretching, Yoga, Tai Chi or Qi Gong
- ◆ Drumming and rhythmic use of musical instruments
- ◆ Mindfulness activities
- ◆ Being in nature
- ◆ Engaging one of the five senses (smell, touch, sound, taste, feel) to bring you into your body and the present moment (i.e., drinking warm tea, mindfully eating)

"Coloring Paper, Markers and Pens" and "She Hums All the Way to the Center": Using Bottom-Up Strategies to Regulate

Teacher Leticia knows this parent meeting might be filled with intense emotions. So, she sets up, in the middle of the table, **coloring paper, markers and pens** and a bin of fidget objects (rubrics cube, fun fidget toys). She puts a tea kettle out with warm water, tea and biscuits. She is aware that when we can fidget, color or draw, and have a nice pot of warm tea and biscuits, that this may regulate the stress system. She also has gentle calming music playing in the background.

Teacher Aracely knows that she is driving to work Monday morning having had a very stressful weekend personally. She feels dysregulated, unrefreshed and her thoughts are, "I don't want to go to work today." She feels a slight headache and low energy in her body. When she drives to work, **she hums all the way to the center** the song "Ave Maria." The Ave Maria reminds her of her grandmother and how that song used to comfort her in times of stress when Abuelita would sing it (relational regulation). By humming it all the way to work, when she arrived, she felt an overarching sense of calm inside her body and a thought, "you got this."

Reflection/Discussion Questions
- ◆ Have you used a bottom-up approach to calm your activated stress response system? Can you list an example?

◆ Have you used a bottom-up approach to regulate yourself and/or co-regulate a family? Which one? What happened as a result?

Intentional disengagement approaches: "Proactive intentional disengagement to regulate and calm"[1] (Perry, 2020c). Intentional disengagement approaches to regulation are the most common way that we as humans regulate and calm ourselves when we are impacted by stress. Disengagement is essentially when a person's brain temporarily, or for longer periods, withdraws from focusing on the external (outside) world and takes a break from thinking. During this time of pause, people can begin to restore their energy. It is as if the antidote of too much thinking/perseverating or focusing on a problem is to take a break mentally to restore your energy. Examples of Intentional Disengagement Regulation strategies include:

◆ Daydreaming or mind-wandering, star-gazing
◆ Disengaging/tuning out for brief moments during a meeting (e.g., to think about how what you are hearing relates to you/your life)
◆ Guided imagery
◆ Prayer or meditation
◆ To "lose oneself" in reading, theater, watching TV, doing art, baking, taking a shower or bath, baking or picking weeds/gardening

"The Lost Herself in Reading": Using Intentional Disengagement Strategies to Regulate

Teacher Fatima takes the bus home after a long and stressful day working with infants and toddlers. Right before she left, another teacher called her out and lectured her about not following a procedure correctly. As she stood in the rain waiting for the bus, she felt very on edge and irritated. Her mind was racing with thoughts such as, "I am such a bad teacher. I don't even know why I am doing this work." During her 40-minute bus drive home, she pulled out her novel and **she lost herself in reading**. Her racing thoughts temporarily dissipated. By the time she reached her home she felt calmer and more regulated. Reading her novel gave Fatima's brain a break from her racing thoughts and allowed some time for her to disengage from her stress. The reading of her novel was a strategy she used to "shut off" her racing mind (intentional disengagement). She arrived home to her older children having cooked dinner, set the table and she heard the laughter and felt the warmth in her home (relational regulation).

Reflection/Discussion Questions

◆ Can you recall a time in your life when your brain felt full, overwhelmed by too much sustained focal attention or too much stress? Have you ever tried an "intentional disengagement approach" to refresh your brain? Can you describe the strategy you used and how you felt after?

Programs, Schools and Organizations Are Impacted by State-Based Functioning Too

All decision-making is state dependent, and you want somebody to be regulated and you want them to have full access to their cortex when they make their decisions… Your job is to make the working environment where they make decisions safer and more regulated and give them opportunities for self-regulating activity and make sure that the policies and practices of the organization and your leadership style are regulated.

(Perry 2020b)

In trauma-responsive environments, strategies are actively and intentionally used to support adults, families and children to maintain emotional and behavioral regulation. Stress related behaviors and dysregulation are met with relational support and activities that tap into core regulatory networks to calm and de-escalate people's bodies and brains. Perry recommends several "organizational care" strategies that support people and organizations to be regulated:

- ◆ **Build in short regulation breaks throughout the workday.** In working with families, the more stress early childhood providers are experiencing, the more frequently they will need short regulation breaks throughout the day and before meeting with a family, especially prior to conversations that may be challenging. Short regulation breaks—from 30 seconds to 5 minutes—when used intentionally and proactively can keep the cortex "open for business" so early childhood staff can reflect, be patient and interact with families during difficult conversations without becoming reactive and to have the capacity to co-regulate parents and family members when they are in a dysregulated state. Short regulation breaks can be as simple as a body stretch, a deep belly breath, going to make a cup of tea, washing your hands, listening to a minute of music, or saying a mantra, prayer or quote to yourself. One example of taking intentional breaks would be during a parent conference day. Instead of scheduling meetings back-to-back, allowing yourself to have 5–15 minutes in between each meeting would allow you to engage in a short regulation activity so you are able to participate in the meeting with the full range of your cognitive and social-emotional capacities.

- ◆ **Decrease the number of decisions people have to make on a given day or during one meeting.** When early childcare providers have to make too many decisions at once, decision fatigue can set in (Perry, 2020b). What does this mean? They have less ability to utilize the full range of the cognitive abilities in their cortex such as reasoning, problem-solving, empathy and self-regulation which may translate into less thoughtful and more reactive decision-making. By simply reducing the number of decisions people have to make (and/or engaging them in regulatory activities just before they need to make those decisions), the cognitive load on adults is reduced and they are more capable of having good judgment and more renewed mental energy to be able to make sound and empathy driven decisions.

Imagine an early childhood program planning to roll out a new attendance policy that will impact the families in the program. A meeting is scheduled to share with parents the new policy and procedures. Knowing this change will require families to complete additional paperwork in a short period of time, this meeting is sure to be filled with parents who become upset. The teacher leading the meeting is very anxious and shares this with her supervisor. Her supervisor understands the neurobiology of stress and she schedules a supervision meeting with the teacher right before the parent meeting. They practice/role play how the meeting will go, then they go for a short walk with each other before the meeting starts. The supervisor provided co-regulatory relational support by being a listener and sounding board and a short walk together as movement can regulate the reactive part of the brain (somato-sensory) so the teacher would have more access to her cortex before the meeting begins.

◆ **Match stakes of decision-making with the length of regulation breaks.** There is a direct relationship between the importance/complexity and stakes associated with decisions and the amount of time needed to regulate beforehand so adults are able to access their cortex. The bigger, more consequential or complex a decision that an individual or group needs to make, the longer amount of time people will need just prior to the decision for a break to engage in regulation strategies. Perry (2020b) describes this as "dosing" decision-making. And conversely, important decisions should not be made when people are least likely to be in a regulated state (e.g., just before lunch or at the end of the day when they are hungry or tired or when they are highly stressed).

Consider an Executive Director (ED) of an early childhood agency runs into the Enrollment Specialist (ES) in the break room at the end of the day. The ED, at 4:45 pm, starts up a conversation asking about the status of enrollment in one of the under enrolled classrooms. The ES becomes highly dysregulated and reacts with defensiveness as she is interpreting the line of questioning to mean she is not doing her job very well. A trauma-responsive ED would recognize that asking this line of questions 15-minutes before the ES leaves for the day is not the best time to have this type of sensitive conversation. Instead, she would plan to ask her the next morning, she would set a time to talk that worked for the ES and prepare her in advance for some of the questions she may ask during the meeting and the reasons for asking these questions. Doing so would allow the ES to have more time for mental preparation and regulation to be able to handle the complexity of the conversation.

◆ **When people are stressed, reduce their workload.** Because of state dependent functioning, people are not as productive or efficient in doing their work (and they are unable to focus or to learn as efficiently) when they are stressed, especially if their stress response systems are activated over a long period of time which is emotionally and physically exhausting. It is important to anticipate this reduction in efficiency and effectiveness and adjust the expectations for what individuals and groups can accomplish. Giving yourself and others grace and recalibrating expectations in times of stress and adversity prevents or minimizes the chance that people will have feelings of self-doubt, guilt and/or shame.

Picture a site supervisor and her teaching team who are coordinating a holiday event for the children and families attending a faith based childcare program. The site super-visor happens to have a lot of personal stress in her family during this time and she has lost one of her long-term teachers to retirement. They have not yet hired someone new and are using substitutes over the holidays. The Executive Director of the program recognizes the signs of stress in her site supervisor and suggests that the family holiday event, although it is a beautiful idea, might be too much at this time. She offers several suggestions in the spirit of minimizing the pressure on her supervisor. These include bringing in additional staff to support her, canceling the event or finding ways to simplify the event to make it less stressful. In taking time to talk and reflect together, they were able to come up with a solution that felt much more manageable to the site supervisor.

◆ **As stress increases, provide more opportunities for people to partner to accomplish their daily work.** Because stress reduces people's capacity, the more stress adults are managing, the greater the need to create opportunities for people to work in partnership in order to maintain efficiency and effectiveness. Working together, adults can provide one another with relational regulation—acting as buffers for stress—and share responsibilities so they are able to maintain the quality of their work.

One example is with a team of family engagement specialists in an organization. They provide ongoing support and services in the homes of families and act as liaisons to the school, classroom and teachers. Previously, the family engagement specialists communicated that they were feeling stressed and isolated which led to the creation of weekly group supervision meetings which greatly reduced their stress. Having opportunities to partner, to have support and support others, to have time for reflection and dialogue with others, acted as a buffer to reduce their stress, decrease their isolation and allowed them to be more present, restored and engaged in their interactions with families.

◆ **Take time for "mind-wandering" before making major decisions**. It is important not to rush into making major decisions. Adults can engage in all the work our cortex affords us—e.g., hearing different perspectives and ideas, analyzing the benefits and limitations of various solutions etc.—however, it's important to plan time for people to allow their brains to engage in a "mind-wandering" process (time for the mind to sort through and make sense of information) by taking regulation breaks. What does this look like? After thinking and talking through an important decision—go home, go for a walk or run, watch a movie, listen to music, get a night's sleep, eat a healthy breakfast and then return to making the decision. This type of break to regulate and support mind-wandering often makes a critical decision easier to make as information is integrated or synthesized in a manner that brings clarity and insight. Mind-wandering is the opposite of focal attention and serves to give the brain a "break to restore."

One example might be a family in your program experiences the loss of a child's beloved pet. The father called to tell you at the end of your workday, and he asks you for advice on how to talk to his child about this loss. What should we tell her he asked? Before making a big decision at the end of the day such as offering advice, the teacher takes that evening to cook dinner, go for a walk and watch a movie with her family and talk to a good friend. The next day, her mind was clear and she was better able to think of ways to approach the situation and to offer support to the child and family.

Reflection/Discussion Questions
◆ Which top-down approach have you used to regulate?
◆ Which bottom-up approach have you used to regulate?

◆ Do you find these strategies are a part of your daily routine and practice in working with families? If not, what is one small step you can take to add a new strategy to your toolbox to keep yourself regulated?

Note

1 **WARNING:** If you are experiencing dissociative or trauma-related triggers with frequent episodes of dissociation (disorientation to time, your location, where you are or have been, losing sense of time and place and/or memory) or disconnection or out of body experiences please seek a professional. It may not be recommended to use intentional disconnection strategies which may further trigger dissociative states. These Intentional Disengagement Strategies are used for temporary relief when you are having too much stress, too much required focal attention and as a result, shutting down temporarily can help restore energy and one's ability to access the executive brain shortly after an intentional disengagement.

References

Acharya, S., & Shukla, S. (2012). Mirror neurons: Enigma of the metaphysical modular brain. *Journal of Natural Science, Biology and Medicine*, *3*(2), 118–124. doi: 10.4103/0976-9668.101878.

Conkbayier, M. (2017). *Early childhood and neuroscience: Theory, research and implications for practice*. New York, NY: Bloomsbury Academic.

Nicholson, J., Perez, L. & Kurtz, J. (2019). *Trauma-informed practices for early childhood educators: Relationship-based approaches that support healing and build resilience in young children*. New York, NY: Routledge.

Perry, B. (2020a). Understanding state dependent functioning. NN COVID Series 2. Retrieved from https://youtu.be/PZg1dlskBLA.

Perry, B. (2020b). Decision fatigue. NN COVID Series 8. Retrieved from https://youtu.be/Yc-Nv8eqfgM.

Perry, B. (2020c). Understanding regulation. NN COVID Series 5. Retrieved from https://youtu.be/L3qIYGwmHYY.

Porges, S. (2011). *The polyvagal theory: Neurophysiological foundations of emotions, attachment, communication, and self-regulation.* New York, NY: Norton.

3

Foundations of High-Quality Family Engagement

There are many resources that describe foundations of high-quality family engagement practice in early childhood—drawing from various disciplines including early childhood education, family support, infant mental health, early intervention, home visiting and social services among others—intended to inform all programs and systems that serve young children and their families. The word cloud on the following page represents words and phrases drawn from these resources that are used to describe high-quality family engagement.

In early childhood, we are still very much at the beginning of a paradigm shift—moving away from traditional parent involvement towards working with parents and families of young children using a family engagement approach. Although the family engagement resources that currently exist provide valuable descriptions and guideposts for creating more respectful and responsive partnerships with families, they are all missing a critical component: **an explicit integration of the science of trauma and resilience.**

Without knowledge of the neurobiology of trauma and resilience and trauma-responsive practices, early educators will struggle to effectively implement and succeed in their

DOI: 10.4324/9781003127666-4

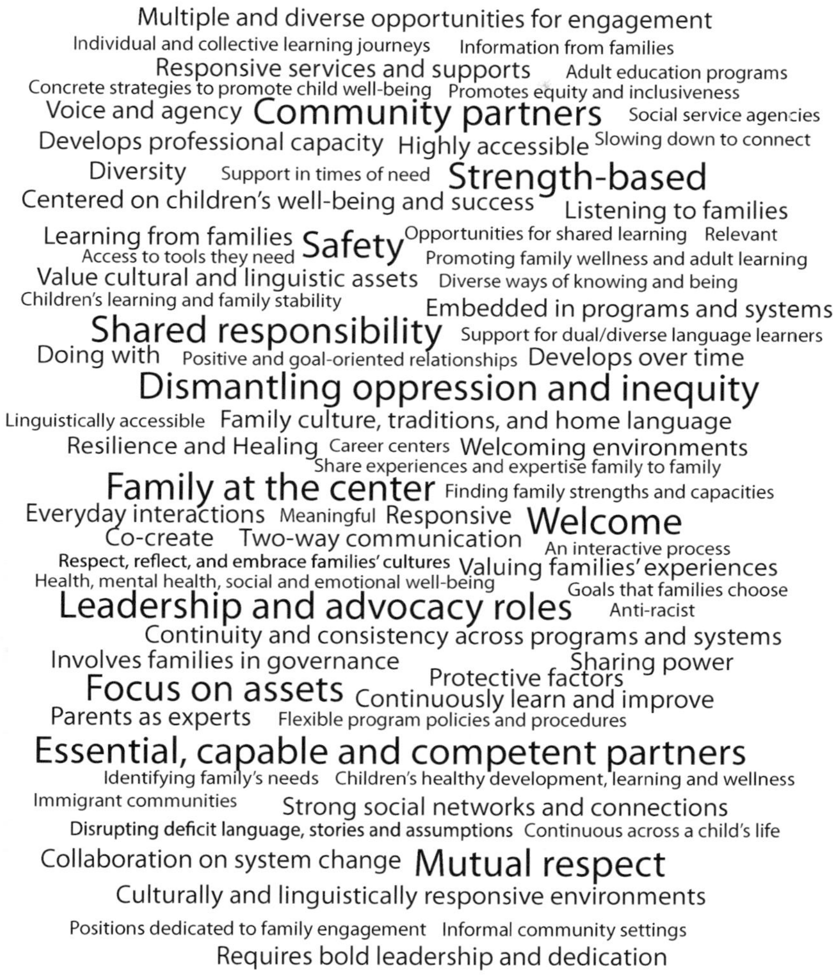

Multiple and diverse opportunities for engagement
Individual and collective learning journeys   Information from families
Responsive services and supports   Adult education programs
Concrete strategies to promote child well-being   Promotes equity and inclusiveness
Voice and agency   Community partners   Social service agencies
Develops professional capacity   Highly accessible   Slowing down to connect
Diversity   Support in times of need   Strength-based
Centered on children's well-being and success   Listening to families
Learning from families   Safety   Opportunities for shared learning   Relevant
Access to tools they need   Promoting family wellness and adult learning
Value cultural and linguistic assets   Diverse ways of knowing and being
Children's learning and family stability   Embedded in programs and systems
Shared responsibility   Support for dual/diverse language learners
Doing with   Positive and goal-oriented relationships   Develops over time
Dismantling oppression and inequity
Linguistically accessible   Family culture, traditions, and home language
Resilience and Healing   Career centers   Welcoming environments
Share experiences and expertise family to family
Family at the center   Finding family strengths and capacities
Everyday interactions   Meaningful   Responsive   Welcome
Co-create   Two-way communication   An interactive process
Respect, reflect, and embrace families' cultures   Valuing families' experiences
Health, mental health, social and emotional well-being   Goals that families choose
Leadership and advocacy roles   Anti-racist
Continuity and consistency across programs and systems
Involves families in governance   Sharing power
Focus on assets   Continuously learn and improve
Parents as experts   Flexible program policies and procedures
Essential, capable and competent partners
Identifying family's needs   Children's healthy development, learning and wellness
Immigrant communities   Strong social networks and connections
Disrupting deficit language, stories and assumptions   Continuous across a child's life
Collaboration on system change   Mutual respect
Culturally and linguistically responsive environments
Positions dedicated to family engagement   Informal community settings
Requires bold leadership and dedication

FIGURE 3.1
Word cloud
Source: Hannah Shack

family engagement efforts. This is because the goals of family engagement—e.g., building trusting relationships, inviting families to share power in reciprocal partnerships, and encouraging parents to engage in collaborative discussions and problem-solving among others—are significantly compromised when adults are experiencing chronic stress and/or impacted by trauma. Therefore, we believe that it is essential that all early childhood professionals learn about trauma and trauma-responsive practice and that family engagement approaches are adapted to incorporate this information.

Early childhood professionals do not need to know if someone experienced trauma or what their trauma history is to use trauma-responsive practices. They just need to recognize what stress-related behaviors look like and the simple steps they can take to support themselves and others to feel safe and be guided back to regulation. Like Su Mei mentions below, just listening to a family or linking them to services is being trauma-responsive and healing engaged.

> We don't have to really know the trauma a family has experienced in order to support them. I think teachers have that misconception that they can't use trauma-informed strategies because they aren't trained therapists. So we need to really emphasize, it's not only for certified therapists, it is also for people like me. We don't need to know the history of the family or be trauma experts. These strategies are good for all families so we just need to understand them and use them. It could be as simple as just being there to listen to a family with the open mindset or linking a family with an important community resource.
>
> (Su Mei Wu, Quality Improvement Coach, BANANAS Resource and Referral Agency)

Core Principles of Trauma-Responsive Practice

Core Principles provide a broad set of values and beliefs that guide early childhood professionals who work with parents and families. We introduce readers to eight Core Principles that we recommend they use to guide their ongoing efforts to build more trauma-responsive, resilience building and healing centered approaches to engaging with young children and their families. These principles are aligned with the most widely cited frameworks for trauma-informed systems of care for children and families and trauma-informed approaches in child serving systems including education and child welfare (e.g., Dorado, Martinez, McArthur & Leibovitz, 2016; National Council for Behavioral Health, 2015). **Our principles were designed specifically with the early childhood field in mind.** We make visible how family engagement "best practices" can be revised to align with the science on toxic stress, trauma, and resilience and the current realities of parents and families of young children today. We briefly list the principles below and discuss each in more depth in the following chapters:

- ◆ Build mutually respectful and trusting relationships that lead to power-sharing partnerships
- ◆ Understand stress and trauma
- ◆ Acknowledge systems of privilege and oppression and take actions to disrupt inequity
- ◆ Reinforce messages of safety and predictability
- ◆ Focus on strengths and assets
- ◆ Provide opportunities for agency and control
- ◆ Use culturally, linguistically and individually responsive practices
- ◆ Intentionally promote coping, resilience and healing

CORE PRINCIPLE: Build Trusting Relationships That Lead to Power-Sharing Partnerships

When parents and families have relational support, they develop important coping skills and resilience. Parents and families thrive in the context of consistent, nurturing and responsive relationships. When we build relationships that are attuned and compassionate, we strengthen trusting connections with others that buffer stress and support coping, healing and wellness. Attuned relationships are responsive versus reactive, engaged versus disengaged and intentionally offer reflective opportunities to promote self-awareness and self-regulation as foundations for empathy, responsiveness and equity.

A trauma-responsive approach to family engagement is first and foremost one that values, invests in and emphasizes the importance of building consistent, trusting and attuned relationships with parents and families. There is an inherent understanding that learning, development, coping, building resilience and healing takes place in the context of consistent, trusting relationships. Children, parents and families must have a felt sense (an inner feeling) of trust and safety in early learning programs. Yet, many individuals with histories of trauma develop internal working models of the world as unsafe—reinforced by bodily sensations, emotions, thoughts and perceptions/expectations—that interfere with their ability to develop trust in relationships or to feel safe in an environment. For this reason, the central focus of relationship building in trauma-responsive environments is **re-building trust** by creating a felt sense of safety.

Safety is reinforced when relationships are based in respect, reciprocity and responsiveness. We draw on Barrera and Kramer's (2009) powerful work in describing the importance of respect, reciprocity and responsiveness as the base for the type of relationships we want to build with parents and families.

Respect: "Differences Do Not Make People Wrong"

We communicate with respect when:

> We believe that the behaviors others exhibit are the result of competent problem-solving given their knowledge and life experience within a particular situation, rather than the result of faulty or incompetent problem-solving or of not knowing what we know. Respect starts with the premise that differences do not make people wrong—they just make them different. This is not to say that we cannot or should not invite change or that all

behaviors are equally life supporting and fully adaptive to a given environment. It is to say that to be respectful, we must first acknowledge the other person's resources, strengths and ability to learn. Respect neither requires nor communicates agreement. It must simply communicate acknowledgement of the legitimacy of the ways others have crafted their lives in response to perceived and learned choices within particular circumstances. Respect acknowledges differences without being judgmental.

(Barrera & Kramer, 2009, pp. 39–41)

Laura Rivas, Family Engagement Specialist, Berkeley Unified School District, describes how this concept of respect is central to her work with families:

I think an essential part of this job is relationship building for many, many reasons. And yet, this work is really tricky and there is no straightforward answer of how to do so. If you're trying to teach literacy, one could say, "this is a strategy you can use and you'll get results." But relationship building just takes time. And sometimes for teachers, it's really frustrating because there are real challenges like not having enough time and not being able to reach families and sometimes there are language barriers and cultural differences. Having a background in community organizing has really helped me to under-stand my relationship to families from a **perspective of solidarity building and community building.** The rela-tionship between me and that family is part of a larger context of anti-racism, fighting homophobia, fighting sexism, fighting systems where communities of color are overrepresented, especially in the carceral (jail/prison) system. Building relationships with that understanding really helps me to have empathy for families in a way that's not sympathy like, "Oh, I feel sorry for them" but instead, to have empathy, acknowledging and recog-nizing the insurmountable factors that families have to face and how they have come to make certain decisions

for their children that we may not understand or that
we might not agree with. Having empathy is necessary
because often what happens is that we jump to judgment
and that really is a big barrier to building meaningful
relationships that support children's success in school
and in life.

Laura draws on her background in community organizing
and her understanding of historical oppression disproportionately impacting People of Color to guide her approach. For
Laura, building relationships with parents and families is akin
to solidarity building and community building—historical and
contemporary movements to dismantle structural racism and
other forms of oppression that disproportionately impact Black,
Indigenous and People of Color. By acknowledging how the
families she works with have been historically and continue
to be minoritized and marginalized within the structures and
systems of our society, Laura acknowledges how the families'
lives outside the walls of the school influence their experiences
within the school. She positions herself as an ally to the families'
struggles and understands that part of communicating "respect"
is honoring every person's unique role in the ongoing fight for
racial and economic justice.

Another example of *respect* is seen with Jenje Dennis, a
toddler teacher working within a program that promotes family
reunification for families impacted by various types of relational
trauma—e.g., deportation, incarceration etc.—within a large
public school district. Jenje describes how part of her work is to
visit families in their homes. She reinforces how easy it is for all
of us to see families impacted by trauma through deficit. Jenje
explains why it is so essential that we scan for strengths and we
acknowledge that much of the trauma many of the families we
are working with face, is the result of systemic and institutional
oppression and injustice:

> I'm a Black American woman with dreadlocks who is
> able to speak Spanish in a community that is Latinx. Our
> community has been really hit with a lot of traumatic

experiences. Our classroom is on a campus where women are coming from an incarcerated situation and also being court ordered to be there. And this is a sanctuary city, so a lot of our families do not feel safe with people coming to their house because of their status. So, I try to connect with the families by using their language. We also focus on the child as that is something we have in common and care deeply about. It is our point of connection and a common thread that give us purpose. We, as early childhood professionals, have to be very careful when working with trauma-impacted families. Maybe you walk into somebody's home and they have things piled up in a way that you would think, "Hey, that's not really safe." But the reality is that the family only has two bedrooms and there's six or more people living in them. So, they have mattresses and people's things stacked up, side by side. I've seen this a lot in my community, how in a family's culture, they're committed to helping each other. So, there may be something that I will not think is safe going into people's homes as a home visitor. Sometimes it's easy to scan for something negative and I could jump to judgment when, in fact, it's a strength of the community or the family and it's a reflection of their culture. I might have a family whose father got deported and the mother moved with her kids into another family's garage. As a home visitor, I cannot go in there and say, this isn't right. The fact that they are homeless, doubling up with another family, that's a reflection of our societal inequities impacting them. As home visitors, we see evidence of that all the time.

Jenje has years of experience working with children and families as a teacher and home visitor. She reminds us that our first reaction, our initial judgment, our knee jerk inner voice that is critical can be trauma or harm inducing (i.e., criticizing, directing, correcting, shaming, blaming). But when we shift our inner voice to, "What is right with this family? What strengths do I see? How is what I see evidence of the family's cultural beliefs and practices? What do I see that reflects the family's coping skills and forms of resilience?" By asking these questions we can shift from a deficit approach to one that respects families through the use of empathy, kindness, curiosity and relational support.

Reflection/Discussion Questions

◆ Have you ever had an initial voice of judgment about a parent or family (i.e., home, interaction, behavior, parenting skill) and you reacted quickly but in a way that you regret?

◆ Do you have an example of when you moved past that initial voice of judgment (i.e., about their home, a parent-child interaction, their behavior, a parenting skill) and took the time to seek the strengths of that parent or family, how certain behaviors may be a learned survival and coping skill or a result of institutional racism and historical trauma?

Reciprocity: "Diversity Is Always Life Enhancing"

Reciprocity builds on respect and is based on an assumption that

> Diversity is always life enhancing…reciprocity seeks to honor another's "voice" or power as a life-enhancing resource. At its core it is a recognition that the behavior of each person in an interaction is an expression of his or her competence and ability to learn rather than of an inability or refusal to learn…The essence of reciprocity is an attitude of openness to another's diverse perspective (i.e., an attitude of "I don't have all the answers"). Such an attitude leaves room for another's "voice" (i.e., perspective and values) even when it disagrees with one's own. Reciprocity does not require denying that one person has more expertise or knowledge than another in particular areas or that one person has more institutionalized authority. What reciprocity does require is acknowledging and trusting that another's learning is an expression of

different learning rather than deficient learning and thus, is of equal value to one's own…entering into interactions only to give—whether knowledge, support, direction or something else—with no acknowledgement of what others, [including] children, can contribute inhibits not only what we might receive, but also the full potential of what we seek to give…a lack of reciprocity erases respect.

(pp. 43–44)

Reflection/Discussion Questions

♦ Can you think back on a time when you shared an idea or voiced your opinion and it was not heard, not valued, disregarded, dismissed or even criticized? How did this feel?

♦ Reflect on this central idea of reciprocity: "What reciprocity does require is acknowledging and trusting that another's learning is an expression of different learning rather than deficient learning." What thoughts and feelings come up for you?

♦ Can you now think back on a past interaction with a family where you put a pause on your initial judgments and sought instead to be curious, to listen, to try to understand how they feel (giving them an opportunity and the space to have a voice) even if it was different from your own inner voice? How do you think the family felt when you heard them?

Responsiveness: "There Is Always a Third Choice"

Responsiveness begins with a value for connection. At its core, it is a recognition that:

There are always more than two choices…to be responsive is to step outside of an either-or framework…[it] acknowledges that an identified problem occurs within a particular relationship and not in isolation (e.g., Joey's behavior is not solely his problem)…to be responsive to another is to entertain the possibility of connection rather than follow the certainty of separation…to shift focus from what divides to what connects. When we see a behavior or interaction and it seems quite incompatible with what we would like to see, or when we experience things that seem contradictory to our perspectives, being responsive calls us to ask, "where are the connections?" …responsiveness seeks to affirm how differences are joined… by shifting perspectives from a "you and I" perspective to a "we" perspective. Responsiveness also entertains mystery….which requires attending to [people] with "focused attention, patience and curiosity" in order to interact with who they truly are, not who [we] think they are. If we seek only certainty and forget mystery, [people] become frozen within our own categories and labels (e.g., the child with ADHD, the resistant mother). Practitioners are no longer in interaction with them—only with their own ideas about them.

(pp. 46–47)

Reflection/Discussion Questions

Many of us, when we engage with a family in distress, we fee out of control. We feel a sense of urgency to help them, to make a difference, to bring order to the feelings of chaos. But we don'th have to react with that sense of urgency all the time, especially if there is not a "survival emergency." We just need to find opportunities to listen, connect and sit in the unknown with a family as we witness and support their journey toward healing. It is never a straight path with clear directions.

- ◆ Have you ever worked with a family and sat in the unknown and the feeling of uncertainty, but you stayed there present, attuned, attentive and listening as you provided emotional attunement and relational safety to them?
- ◆ Have you been able to trust the process, let go of your first assumptions or attempts to control, direct, actively help and take time to pause and be curious?

Things are not always as they seem if we only look at the surface. Our brain tends to react with simple summaries such as "this child has that behavior because of their parenting skills." When we stop at "it is your fault" we miss the layers and layers of possibilities and solutions. Family engagement means that "we are in this together" not "I need you to change in this way." Family engagement is, as you will see in the vignette below with Muriel, about finding genuine points of connection with families.

"Where do you find that genuine connection to them as a human being?": An example of responsiveness in action— Muriel Johnson, Lead Teacher, Private Preschool Center

> We never know somebody's story. We can always find something to connect with when we are working with a parent or family. **I always ask myself, where can I find that genuine connection to them as a human being?** If we are always thinking that we are so different from them, "There is no way I can relate to these people," well, this type of thinking will disable us from being able to make a connection. I may think that there's nothing that I can relate to but it's not true. For example, I think a lot of times for White people, they have such discomfort around People of Color because it's as if we're alien. And what they know about us, or they think they know us from the movies, media, whatever. But they don't know me. "I'm a classical pianist, why are you talking to me about rap music?" Why? Because people can be stuck in a stereotype of what they think they know about me. But they should be thinking, "This is a human being, what do I notice about her as an individual? Wow, this woman wears beautiful shoes, just like me." If we look at a person as a whole human being, we can always find a place to bridge—to create a connection so we can communicate with them. And as a teacher, you're with their kid. What better point to be able to build a relationship around? We might say, "Your son was singing all day, did he learn that from you? It seems like he loves to sing."

"Oh, his grandma sings to him? Thank you for sharing that with me." The goal is that we find a place to relate to the parent and family. And to make sure that we aren't only connecting with them when there has been a difficult day or to report "He needs more diapers." What is critical is that we are always asking ourselves, what is the content of my communication with this parent? How do I make them feel like I'm invested in their child and that I respect them as a parent and as another human being? A lot of parents bring their kids to centers, but they don't feel a connection with the center or the people there. It's a place for their child to get fed and get cleaned up and take a nap, somewhere relatively safe while they can go to work, but they're not feeling like they're embraced. And yet, every family needs to feel valued and embraced.

Our limbic brain (responsible for relational connections and emotions) is always scanning the environment to answer the question, "Do I belong here? Am I accepted and do I feel safe?" If/when the answer feels like "no," our brain perceives threat and activates our stress response system. Muriel reinforces how important it is that early childhood professionals are always asking ourselves, "how do I make sure that every family feels valued and embraced and my language and actions are sending messages that they belong here and are valued in this program?"

Reflection/Discussion Questions

♦ When you are communicating with a parent or family, what are the small ways (nonverbally or verbally) you show them you are invested in their child, you care about them, they belong and are valued in your program?

Emergent Listening with Families

Trusting relationships are built from what Bronwyn Davies (2014) calls emergent listening. In most of the conversations throughout our day, we "listen in order to fit what we hear into what we already know" (p. 21). We do not expect, and therefore, often we do not allow our underlying worldviews and central beliefs about "the way things are" to be disrupted and rearranged in our day-to- day interactions. Davies calls this *"listening as usual."* In contrast, emergent listening, involves, "opening up the ongoing possibility of coming to see life, and one's relation to it, in new and surprising ways" (p. 21). **Emergent listening is about "being open to being affected" by what one hears someone say, rather than simply responding**. It requires you as a listener to be open to *being changed* by what you hear or experience in your communication and interactions with others, possibly in a fundamental way that challenges your mindset, worldview and/or taken-for granted assumptions and beliefs. This is a deep form of listening that creates opportunities for transformative learning to occur. When we remain open to changing our minds after tuning in to truly listen to someone else and remaining open to whatever we learn as a result, we communicate a powerful message to children and adults that they are seen, heard, respected, validated and safe.

To engage in emergent listening requires self-awareness of our own thoughts, feelings, values, beliefs or judgments in the moment. It demands that we are open to moving beyond our initial reactions and that we are willing to imagine the world through another's perspective, to expand our awareness, to let go of the status quo in the service of increasing our empathy and understanding of others' perspectives. Emergent listening is an aspirational skill—we never master this practice, but instead, we are always striving to strengthen our capacity to engage in it.

Following is an example of a Family Engagement Specialist describing why emergent listening is so central to her process of building trusting relationships with families.

"You're just trying to get me to do this. You're not really trying to hear me": An example of emergent listening in work with families—Laura Rivas, Family Engagement Specialist, Berkeley Unified School District

> I try not to approach people with a set agenda because then the adults feel like, "Okay, **you're just trying to get me to do this. You're not really trying to hear me.** You're not really trying to understand where I'm coming

from." I've heard so many educators I work with say, "I said the right thing. I didn't say anything wrong. I don't understand why they (the parent or family) got so upset." There are so many non-verbal messages we communicate to families in our conversations with them. It's our facial expression, our tone of voice, our eye contact. All of that reflects what we really think or how we feel about that person. So, we might be saying one thing but if we're really feeling "I'm so annoyed that you asked this question" we may be responding with words that answer a parent's question but what they really perceive is that we are bothered by the fact that they're even asking. These things are intangible, but so important for us to become aware of and to become part of our self-reflection. If parents are not feeling heard or not feeling seen, some will just give it to you raw, like here it is, all my anger and frustration whereas some will be at the other end of the spectrum and just shut down and won't respond to your call, not come to any meeting and they just disappear.

Laura recognizes that building a relationship with a family is not about conveying her expert knowledge to them but instead, through being aware and intentional about welcoming non-verbal cues such as body language, facial expressions and voice tones. She reminds us that the verbal and non-verbal cues we send to families can convey a powerful message, "I am here with you, I am listening to what you need and I want to send you every message both verbally and nonverbally that you are safe and valued." Laura understands that emergent listening involves listening to her own feelings and reactions while ensuring that her responses are responsive to the family's needs, not just her own needs.

"Parents will have different relationships with different staff and that is good. The trust should be built across the program"—Chantelle Marin, Lead Teacher, Educare, Omaha

Chantelle Marin, lead teacher at Educare, Omaha, describes that one goal we can have in early childhood programs is to support parents to build relationships with more than one person within our programs. Having multiple people within a program that they can connect with can strengthen families' sense of community, reduce their isolation and allow them to have different types of relationships that serve different purposes. Chantelle explains:

> We are fortunate to have a really interdisciplinary team at our site—classroom teachers, a health coordinator and family support specialist all coming together for the child and the family. I inform the team if I observe something with a child that I may have concerns about and I'm honest about that with the parent. This way the families know that they have multiple people they can come to talk to about their child's experience in our program. A parent might have some things that she only feels comfortable talking to our Family Engagement Specialist about and other things she only feels comfortable talking to me, her child's teacher, about. I have two other teachers in my room and it doesn't mean that all three of us have to have the exact same relationship with that parent. There are some parents that only feel comfortable talking to certain teachers and that's totally fine. We want to meet parents where they're at.

Chantelle helps us understand that building relationships may mean that parents develop varying degrees of trust with different people within our programs and this is OK. We can work on not personalizing when this happens ("Why don't they like me?"), but instead, honoring and acknowledging that having multiple relationships within a program creates a foundation for relational support that is healthy and a stress reducing trauma-responsive practice that we want all families to benefit from.

Reflection/Discussion Questions
  ◆ How do you expand the opportunity for families to build relational connections with more than one person in your program?
  ◆ How does expanding opportunities for families to build relational connections with others help them feel safe?

"Lorena's Story": Putting all the pieces of the trauma-responsive relationship puzzle together—Laura Rivas, Family Engagement Specialist, Berkeley Unified School District

The following vignette is the story of a child named Lorena and how things are not always as they appear on the surface. Laura, a Family Engagement Specialist explains through this story how she takes a trauma-responsive approach to building responsive relationships with Lorena's family using respect, reciprocity, responsiveness and emergent listening. As you read the vignette, look for specific examples of how these concepts are applied in context to build and strengthen trust with Lorena's mother in order to collaborate with her to support Lorena:

> Lorena started kindergarten as a quiet, soft-spoken child. She kept to herself in the beginning, not rushing to make any new friends. For the most part, she listened to her teacher and followed instructions in class the first few days of school. Lorena had a really hard time adjusting to school. On several occasions, she would start crying in the classroom while students were working on an activity together and after a while, she started walking out of the classroom and roaming the hallways. On one occasion, she managed to leave the classroom when the teacher was not looking and hid in the school garden. We were all really scared for what felt like an eternity (about 15 minutes), as we did not know where she was. Lorena's teacher, Ms. Lopez, had tried multiple times to contact her parent, but there was no response to her calls home. Ms. Lopez began to feel frustrated.
>
> "How can they expect me to help if they don't even respond to a phone call?" she asked me.
>
> "Let me try reaching out," I said. "I have some school supplies in my office and I can offer to give a bag to Lorena." I called later that evening and did not get an answer. I thought maybe her parent got home really late from work. The next day I called in the morning. No answer again, so I left a message. I tried texting.

Nothing. That day, I was in the teachers' lounge catching up with Ms. Lopez, letting her know that I had not yet been successful in reaching Lorena's family. Another staff member overheard our conversation and said, "Have you tried reaching out to Lucy? That is her older sister and she is in high school with my daughter. She misses a lot of school, and my daughter says they are all worried about her." I reached out to my colleague at the high school, who got consent to share Lucy's phone number with me. I picked up the phone and called right away. Lucy answered, "Hello?" "Hi, this is Laura. I work at Lincoln Elementary where your little sister goes to school. Do you have a minute to chat?" I always like to check in and see if I'm calling at an OK time. This makes a difference and people feel like you recognize that they have lives and responsibilities, too. "Sure" she responded and I could hear a bit of hesitation in her voice.

I let her know my job at the school was to support families and that we were beginning to worry about Lorena because she seemed really sad all the time, was not interested in making friends and would often say she missed her dad. "My dad died last year," said a shaky voice on the other end of the line. "He died of cancer. Lorena was really close with him." My heart broke for Lorena and her family. At that moment, I realized that none of my family engagement strategies from all the training I attended were going to be useful. The priority was to take the time to listen and get to know this family so that together we could figure out the best way for school staff to support them.

Lorena was enrolled in the after-school program and was at school from 8:00am to 5:30pm when her mother or older sister picked her up. I decided to stay at work late one day and see if I would run into Lorena's family as they picked her up from school. I had the pleasure of meeting Ms. Arias, Lorena's mother. She had a really tough and guarded exterior, although soft-spoken, I could tell it would take time to gain her trust. I met with Ms. Arias several times, offering various different resources for her family. One day it was a bag of school supplies. The next day it was offering to sign her up for a school-based food pantry program. Finally, after several in-person meetings with her, she began to soften up. She also started to answer my calls and slowly, she started to open up about what she and her family had been through. She shared that Lorena was only three and a half years old when her dad passed away. Ms. Arias wanted to protect young Lorena from the heartache of losing her father, so she did not take Lorena to the funeral, and did not tell her that her dad had died for several months. When Ms. Arias finally told Lorena, she did not seem to understand what it meant that her dad had died. Ms. Arias was not able to take any time off work to be with her children, to grieve, or to process all they had been through. She had no choice but to continue working, cleaning other peoples' homes and to make ends meet as the sole breadwinner for her family. Ms. Arias came to the US as an adult, escaping the grips of poverty in her home country. She and her late husband went through the horribly brutal experience of crossing a heavily militarized border, in order to provide better opportunities for their children. Now she was a widow, navigating grief alone, without a close network of family to support her.

After a home visit, where Ms. Arias shared bits and pieces of her life story, and my gentle encouragement for Lorena to see our school counselor, Ms. Arias gave her consent. I am very sensitive when it comes to suggesting therapy or counseling to a parent because it may not be what they need at that moment. In our school staff meetings, we are very quick to jump to the conclusion that children who are experiencing trauma need therapy or counseling. As a trauma survivor, I know first-hand the transformative power of therapy and counseling. However, without addressing the immediate needs that a family is facing, suggesting they go to counseling is basically asking them to put in the work of healing when they may not be ready for it. Healing takes work. I think often we underestimate how much work it actually takes for humans to truly heal trauma wounds. Lorena met with the school counselor, twice a week for the rest of the school year in kindergarten. During that time, I developed a close and caring relationship with Lorena. I would sometimes go to the cafeteria at lunch time, or to the playground during recess just to see how she was doing. Every time she saw me, she would run up and give me a hug.

As the family engagement specialist, I was able to deepen my relationship with Lorena and her family over the years through various home visits, phone calls, in-person check-ins, invitations to several school events and helping to bridge communication with our school staff. Lorena is now in 5th grade and excelling academically. She has developed sweet friendships with peers and has no problem asking for help when she needs it. Ms. Arias called me recently and asked if I could help her with the middle school enrollment process, since it is all online. I realized how far we have come, and the fact that she felt comfortable reaching out to me for support is a huge victory. That is true engagement. It is not a transactional relationship, where school staff try to get families to see from our perspective, but a transformative relationship where we remain open to learning, with humility, and allow ourselves to grow together in supporting the child.

An important aspect of building relationships with families that is often left unsaid, is how much emotional labor it requires from us as early childhood professionals, to understand our own histories and experiences of trauma and to acknowledge that our identities, our personal experiences of privilege and oppression, of being harmed and learning how to cope, build resilience and to heal will absolutely be present in our work with families (a truth that is often invisible and undervalued). It is important to acknowledge this reality and be willing to explore how our own experiences and histories with trauma are both beneficial (helping us to have empathy with families) and potentially problematic (when their stress and trauma is triggering for us) as we work with families. Laura understands these relationships and shares how learning to work responsively with families impacted by trauma is intertwined with her own journey of healing. When we become aware of our own trauma history and cultivate self-awareness, we can better engage with families impacted by trauma. For one, you cannot help anyone farther than you have helped yourself and two, what is out of your conscious awareness can unconsciously drive some of your reactions.

> I have now been serving my community for eight years in my role as Family Engagement Specialist at two elementary schools. When I first started this job, my first-born child was in preschool. I had no idea how my own parenting would be impacted and transformed by this experience. Most of the families I work most closely with, have experienced some form of trauma in their childhood or adult lives. As People of Color, particularly Black and Indigenous, or darker-skinned folks, living and existing in the world at this specific moment in time feels like a constant experience of trauma. Being told over and over again that what you feel, see, hear, the way you are impacted—is not real—is a form of violence. Schools are too often places where these experiences of trauma re-surface, especially if you have not had the opportunity to process what you went through as a child. For parents, this can be a very emotionally vulnerable situation. As a survivor of childhood trauma, I have had to face my own fears as they emerged when my first-born child started school. I have 20 years of experience working with children, youth and families in various supportive capacities, but being a parent to two young children required a whole new level of support, healing and self-reflection.
>
> Laura Rivas

Reflection/Discussion Questions

◆ How did Laura practice respect, responsiveness and reciprocity? Are there examples of how you used this trauma-responsive approach with a parent/family?

◆ How did Laura use emergent listening in the vignette? Can you remember a time you used emergent listening with a parent or family and changed (a belief or behavior) based on what you heard?

◆ Our trauma histories as early childhood professionals come to work with us and influence how we show up. How can you be aware of your trauma history and its impact on you while relating to families, hearing them and building positive relationships with them?

References

Barrera, I., & Kramer, L. (2009). *Using skilled dialogue to transform challenging interactions: Honoring identity, voice, and connection* (1st ed.). Baltimore, MD: Brookes Publishing.

Davies, B. (2014). *Listening to children: Being and becoming.* London: Routledge.

Dorado, J., Martinez, M., McArthur, L. & Leibovitz, T. (2016). Healthy environments and response to trauma in schools (HEARTS): A whole-school, multi-level, prevention and intervention program for creating trauma-informed, safe and supportive schools. *School Mental Health, 8,* 163–176. doi.org/10.1007/s12310-016-9177-0.

National Council for Behavioral Health. (2015). Retrieved from www.thenationalcouncil.org/wp-content/uploads/2016/07/Trauma-Sensitive-Schools-webinar-10-19-15.pdf.

4

CORE PRINCIPLE: Understand Stress and Trauma

Many parents and families have experienced trauma. Understanding the prevalence of trauma and the long-term impact it has on individuals, families and communities in one or more life-domains (socially, emotionally, mentally, physically and spiritually) is important and allows educators to create more inclusive and trauma-responsive environments. Understanding how stress and trauma can affect children, families, communities and organizations can help to reframe otherwise confusing or frustrating behavior. This includes learning about impacts on relationships, communication and learning. It also means using this knowledge to inform policies, procedures, practices and intervention plans with a goal of creating more compassionate, strength-based and empathy-based interactions and support for children and families impacted by trauma instead of re-traumatizing and/or causing them further harm.

Understanding the impact of stress and trauma and their impact on learning, development and human functioning is central to

DOI: 10.4324/9781003127666-5

a trauma-responsive approach. Trauma (past or present) leaves individuals feeling a complete loss of control and can have a long-term impact on the way they perceive interactions, the environment and/or events in the world. Stress and trauma can adversely impact our relational connections, our feelings of safety, our ability to trust and our capacity to cope in the face of challenges and adversity. However, trauma does not and should not define any of us. Maintaining hope, developing resilience, using our sources of strength and wisdom all help us to rewire our brains throughout our lifespans and to reduce any short- or long-term impacts of the adversities we face. Understanding the neurobiology of stress and trauma will help early childhood professionals to create programs and implement family engage-ment strategies that move from trauma-inducing towards trauma-informed and ideally, to trauma-responsive and healing centered environments. As Siegel and Bryson (2015) state,

> We are not held captive for the rest of our lives by the way the brain works at this moment—we can actually rewire it so we can be healthier and happier. This is true not only for children and adolescents, but also for each of us across the life span.
>
> (p. 1)

Understanding Stress and Trauma can mean listening to a parent when they are upset and trying to find a way to give them a voice to share their concerns. When we listen instead of being reactive, and we look below the surface of the behavior to try to understand the message a parent is trying to communicate to us, only then can we help them feel respected and promote healing. The following vignette provides one window into what this can look like in our work with families.

"You care about your daughter. Sometimes we get upset when things aren't going right."—Shawn M. Bryant, Founding Director and Chief Learning Officer at Teaching Excellence Center

> Last year I was working with the YMCA and helping at one of their preschool sites. One of the mothers I worked

closely with had a child enrolled in one of the Head Start classrooms and her 4½ year old child, Bri, was on the Autism Spectrum and had almost no expressive language. Bri would have outbursts and she stopped resting during naptime. Staff had to sit with her in the yard while other children would rest. As her behavior escalated, Bri started pushing over furniture in the class-room. Everyone believed these were displays of her frus-tration as she was not able to engage in play with her peers. Bri rode the bus each day and spent half of her mornings in a public-school inclusion classroom and the other half with the Head Start program. When I began meeting with Bri's mother, she was upset. She kept telling me, "You all are trying to kick my daughter out again." I knew the Family Advocates had been listening to her, the Assistant Directors had been listening to her, the Mental Health Consultant was listening to her. They were all listening to her and among themselves thinking, "how can we deescalate this mother? She's in the hallway and she's raising her voice. What can we do to calm her down?" I took a different approach. I didn't ask her to lower her voice. I knew why she was raising her voice. She thinks we're going to kick her kid out of the program. She believes that raising her voice is going to get her heard. She's upset. I simply said, "Please sit down beside me." She sat down next to me. And my first comment was, "You're supposed to be upset." She looked at me and she kind of reared back. I said, **"You care about your daughter. Sometimes we get upset when things aren't going right."** I could literally feel her body change. Her shoulders began to rest. Her chin went down and her eye gaze shifted, now she was looking directly at me. To me, this is family engagement, not just meeting someone where they are, but mirroring to them, "this is what you brought," and then being intentional about my response. I did not respond to her by saying, "You're wrong, lower your voice. I want to call the police. I can't talk to you until you calm down." None of that would be helpful to her or to me. She needed to have a felt sense that she was being heard. She needed to hear me say back to her, "You think we are trying to kick your daughter out of the program" even if what we were intending to communicate was, "We think you need to have another IEP meeting so we can get your daughter some additional services." By supporting this mother to feel heard, I was able to build trust with her and to shift her mindset from, "They're working against me. They're blaming me." to "They're working with me." Because I understand how stress impacts adults' thinking and behavior, I understood what story this mother's words and actions were communicating to us and what she needed in that moment to feel heard and respected. Focusing on building trust with her led to an important shift in our conversations together. Once she no longer worried that we were trying to kick her daughter out of the program, we could focus on talking through an important question together: How can we work together to better meet Bri's needs?

Shawn's story shows us that by supporting Bri's mother to feel heard, he was able to build trust and shift this mom's feeling from "everyone is working against me" to "they are working with me." When Shawn was able to respond using his understanding of stress and trauma, he moved his own inner voice from "what is wrong with you?" to a trauma-responsive inner voice that instead asks, "what is your behavior communicating to me?" This shifts his energy to mobilizing trauma-responsive strategies to help this mother feel a sense of safety through his actions including listening, curiosity, staying calm and looking past her words to try to understand and empathize with her underlying concerns.

Reflection/Discussion Questions

◆ Like Shawn, have you ever found yourself engaging with a parent and you had a shift in your inner voice from "what is wrong with you" to "I wonder what your behavior is communicating to me about what you need and/or want to express right now?" How did that different perspective change how you responded to the parent?

The following vignette highlights another example of an early childhood professional using his understanding of stress and trauma to support a child and family to feel safety and support. Jonathan Iris-Wilbanks, a Certified Child Life Specialist, who works with children and families in hospital settings is continually reading the body language of the families he works with to look for signs of stress, and when he sees stress-related behaviors, he takes intentional actions to reassure and to help them feel safety and as sense of control. Jonathan understands that by helping parents to decrease their stress levels, they will be better able to co-regulate their children to feel calm, regulated and safe.

"I really spend a lot of time with families thinking about their stress level because that just goes right into the child's little body"—Jonathan Iris-Wilbanks, Certified Child Life Specialist

"I'm always taking the temperature or thinking about the parents and families I work with, What is their body telling me about how stressed they are right now?" I look for parents or family members who are showing body cues of stress like clenched hands or folded arms or they're holding onto their child's bed and their body is saying, "Don't take this person from me." These messages are important information for me. Before I start talking to the parent, I position my body so I'm not blocking the doorway and I'm not hovering over them. I think to myself, "Can I go get a chair and sit down to be at the parent's level before we even start talking?" I try to neutralize the things that are stressful for the parent and send the message, "I'm a person in this environment who's going to listen to you." I might ask the parent, "Do you want to talk alone for a moment away from your kiddo?" If they consent to having a private conversation I can ask them, "How are you doing in this moment? What has been the most stressful for you? Do you feel like people are listening to you?" I open up a space for parents to tell me about interactions they are having in the hospital. Or sometimes, they say things like, "I don't know where my car is parked. We came in the middle of the night to the emergency department and I just straight up don't know where my car is." And so I ask for their consent to offer support, "Can I walk with you to the parking garage to help you find your car?" Sometimes it's just something like that. Nobody in this environment is typically asking, what are the needs of this family right now?

I'm always trying to get a feeling for how stressed somebody is or if there are words or actions that are really stressing them out that we can address. They might not have slept. They might not have eaten. Maybe the parents are worried because they don't know how the older brother is going to get to school that day. They might have their own traumas from when they were young and this is triggering all of that or a past experience in a hospital where somebody had a bad outcome or didn't live. And now all of that is flooding back in at this moment. Maybe their child only has an ingrown toenail and their stress reaction really doesn't match, but it doesn't matter. If the stress is there, it needs to be addressed. I think to myself, how is this person coping? Are they coping? What is their body telling me? Somebody who's very, very stressed needs to hear something a number of times before they understand it so I might need to repeat what I'm saying. Or I might give them the opportunity to take a break, a chance to take notes or to think of questions that they're thinking of so they don't forget them when the doctor comes around. **I really spend a lot of time with families thinking about their stress level because that just goes right into the child's little body**. So, I feel like if I can help a parent or caregiver be a little less stressed and a little more empowered in that space, the child will benefit. Once I listen to the parent and understand what their worries and needs are, I can be responsive.

How Is the Principle Understanding of Stress and Trauma Reflected in This Vignette?

◆ Jonathan pays attention to all the stress reactions by looking for clues in the parents' and family members' bodies.

◆ He offers them opportunities to take notes or take a break so they can continue to regulate their own bodies and engage their thinking brain.

◆ He understands the power differential of entering a place that automatically makes the parents feel powerless or out of control and he takes intentional actions to reduce the power differential and relate to parents in a manner that positions them with voice, choice and agency.

Reflection/Discussion Questions

◆ When working with families, in what ways do you consider the various cues they send (what Jonathan describes as "observing the temperature") about their stress levels? Can you give an example of a family you worked with who showed clues about their states of stress in the following areas: body sensations (face, shoulders, hands/arms, eyes etc.)? Voice tone, intonation, rhythm of the words? Feelings they expressed? Behaviors you observed?

◆ When you observe signs of stress (body, posture, facial expressions, voice tone, behavior), what steps or strategies do you take to help a parent or family feel safe or to provide them with more control in a situation?

Working with families and communities experiencing toxic and traumatic stress calls for an understanding of stress and trauma. When we enter a family's home, we too might sense the traumatic stress they are experiencing. This can trigger us to feel like we want to take control and do something which can lead early childhood staff to be directive or give expert advice with the hope of making an impact. As you read the vignette below, you can see that it is the opposite that is needed. Imparting our expert knowledge is not the trauma-responsive strategy that will make a difference. Valentina Torres, an early childhood mental health specialist, understands it is scanning for strengths, listening, being curious and allowing space for parents and families to talk is the most trauma-responsive and healing approach we can take. These are the practices that lead to building a positive relationship and sense of trust with families.

"First hear where they are, listen to their story and move from there and really try and come at it from a strength-based perspective"—Valentina Torres, Early Childhood Mental Health Specialist, Jewish Family and Children's Services

> As a mental health clinician, I provide social and emotional support to staff, administration, children and parents/families in different preschools and early childhood settings. I also receive referrals for children who are identified as having challenges including trauma-related behaviors. My role as a clinician is to begin a dialogue with the child's family and explore options for possible treatment for the child and/or the family to address the presenting concerns.
>
> A lot of the families I work with live in very traumatic situations, households and communities with a lot of unresolved trauma, trauma that they themselves have never really processed or even had an opportunity or the privilege of addressing because they just needed to move forward to survive. Over the years I have learned that the best way to engage with them is not to force them into any therapy or intervention, but instead, to **first hear where they are, listen to their story and move from there and really try and come at it from a strength-based perspective**. When I initially meet with a family I take the time to get to know them. I ask questions like "Where are you from? What languages do you speak? What was your childhood like? What is going well in your family? What activities do you enjoy doing as a family? What brings you comfort in times of stress? What is it like to ask for help? How would you like me to provide

feedback to you?" I find that asking questions like these helps families feel at ease; it allows them to tell me about themselves by focusing on their abilities and strengths. Families are in such a vulnerable position when seeking mental health services, usually something isn't going the way they planned. So, I believe it is important to acknowledge this but to also to bring in what is going right. So I focus on creating rapport with the family and showing them that I am someone who is trustworthy. By asking questions about them, I am showing them that I care, that I will listen to them, that I respect them and that I want our relationship to be a collaboration. These kinds of questions also encourage the family to reflect and it deepens their awareness of what might be going on for their child.

Oftentimes, when I talk to parents and families who don't know what early childhood mental health is or what it's about, they will say, "But they're just so little, how can anything be wrong?" Or sometimes they will say, "Here's my child, fix him or her" and they will drop them in my lap and assume I will make everything better. And so part of my job is taking some time to let the families understand that oftentimes the children's behavior really has roots in how they understand and feel about what is going on in the family, unresolved traumas, the things that they experienced but can't make any sense of because nobody wants to talk to them about it or they don't know how to. I believe it is important for parents to understand how their children experience trauma. One of the ways we can do this is by listening to children and observing how they play. For example, during one session, a child started crashing the toy cars and screaming, and his parents were embarrassed and started to scold him. In that moment, I gently sat closer to the parent and I inquired about how they were feeling in that moment. By increasing their awareness to their own internal state, I can help calm them. Then I said to the child, "those cars are crashing and it sounds very loud and scary." This helps name the feeling behind the behavior for both the parent and the child. Then, I can connect the current emotional response that the parents and child are having to when they witnessed a car crash outside their house. In the play with the child, I can then ask if there are any helpers we can bring in to help the cars. This can bring in for the child the idea that scary things happen but there are people who can help. If the child can't think of a helper I can ask the parents and they can join in the play as a helper and the parent and child can have a reparative experience. In a later session, I could explain to the parent how reenacting an experience is normal for children who have witnessed a traumatic event and that by providing space for them to play it out safely, we can help them make sense of what happened. I might also tell parents that their own emotional response is important to notice and tend to. Paying attention to their feelings and calming themselves is an important first step in helping their children regulate.

A lot of the families that I work with are Latino and 80% of the work that I do is in Spanish. So there's a lot of trauma related to getting to the United States. Just the mere fact of getting here is traumatic. The things that they've lived through and experienced, almost always the reasons they are coming here is because they've lived through a lot of things in their home country. They are escaping kidnappings, killings, gangs and drug wars. And then they travel here and it's rough. They share a lot of stories of dehydration and fainting and crawling through things, rape and torture. I hear a lot about violence around money: holding people for money, doing things for money. And then they get here and there's a really negative view of immigrants. And so they arrive and then they don't speak the language and there is a lot of acculturation trauma that can happen just settling here. And most of the work that I do is out in East Oakland and that in and of itself is a neighborhood that has experienced a lot of trauma.

As an early childhood professional, we feel better when we can help, fix and offer solutions. It feels uncomfortable to just sit with a family and listen to their story without offering advice. But every piece of advice that comes from us can result in sending underlying messages that what they are doing is wrong. When we listen and help uncover their sources of strength, wisdom and cultural ways of knowing, we can reinforce their feelings of safety, messages that we see their strengths and capacities which we can build upon to strengthen their regulation and to develop a trusting relationship. When another adult begins to trust you then that is where the true healing can begin. Families will be more likely to listen, be a thinking partner and to access the executive brain (cortex) where they can find their own solutions. This is what Valentina shows us and she helps us understand the trauma-responsive principle in action: Understanding Stress and Trauma, acknowledging the impact of trauma in a family's life and the power of listening and respectful relationships to support healing.

Family Engagement work requires that we understand stress and trauma (and state dependent functioning) for adults and for children. In the following vignette, we see how being trauma-responsive is about recognizing triggers in children and adults, seeking to understand the meaning underneath the behavior and how we can move from being reactive to being responsive by using strategies to create feelings of safety and support.

"We kept saying to him, 'That's Emma's mom' but he didn't stop shaking"—Kathryn Clark Silveira, Owner/Operator of CARE4EM Family Child Care (Cultivating A Responsive Environment for children, parents, teachers, caregivers, all of EM)

> One of our parents works for the Vallejo police department. And she came to the preschool classroom in the middle of the day to drop something off while she was in her uniform. And one of our young Black boys, Terrell, saw her uniform and just started shaking. He sees this mom all the time in her regular clothes but did not recognize her that day and had a strong triggering response when he saw the uniform. **We kept saying to him,**

"That's Emma's mom" but he didn't stop shaking. We rubbed his back; we took some deep breaths with him and we told him over and over that he was safe, that we would take care of him and that the police officer was not here for us but was dropping off a package at the preschool. I called Emma's mother that evening, shared what happened and asked if she could refrain from wearing her uniform when coming into the classroom. Emma's mother was very open and responsive to this request and said next time she will come out of uniform and if that is unavoidable, she would call in advance to make an arrangement that would help Terrell feel safe (i.e. drop off or pick up outside). I also spoke with Terrell's mother and explained what happened, how Terrell responded and the different ways we tried to help him feel safe again ("I was able to rub his back. He used his breathing and then went outside and he rode on the bike").

Kathryn and the staff acknowledged how Terrell's body was associating the police uniform with his lived experiences as a young Black boy. She worked with the adults and Terrell to create an environment where Terrell could feel safe and not have to experience that traumatic trigger again.

As we learned in this vignette, Understanding Stress and Trauma also means observing children and families and their patterns of trauma reminders or trauma triggers. When we understand what triggers a child or parent (i.e., activates their stress response system), we can eliminate or remove a trigger or prepare children/adults in advance for when that event will be coming so that they don't respond with alarm. In doing so, we help them feel safe.

Reflection/Discussion Questions

- ♦ Thinking of the trauma-responsive principle, Understanding Stress and Trauma, have you worked with a child and took steps to either eliminate a trigger in the environment or to prepare a child in advance before the triggering event took place? How did you communicate with the parent or family about this trigger to seek their input and/or their expert advice about strategies to use to reduce stress and reinforce safety for the child?

Valendena Koneck-Wilcox, a Family Engagement Specialist for Educare, Omaha, highlights how Understanding Stress and Trauma is not only for individual early childhood educators but also for programs and organizations to embed in their policies and practices. In a typical day she observes lots of stress-related—fight, flight, freeze—behaviors in her work with parents and families and with staff. As a result, she is absorbing their stress and must be very intentional so she does not meet their dysregulated energy with her own. Instead, she works hard to remain calm, co-regulate and guide others back to regulation. How does she keep herself energized, refreshed, focused and calm? Having a supervisor who understands the impact of stress and trauma on adults' behavior and working within an agency that has created structures to provide support to staff to regulate their thoughts and strong emotions. Valendena explains in the vignette below the important difference it makes to have organizational support.

"I'm able to vent without a filter"—Valendena Koneck-Wilcox, Family Engagement Specialist, Educare, Omaha, Nebraska

> Recently, after a phone call with a parent who yelled at me, I went into my boss's office and I said, "I need to just talk this out. I'm not looking for advice. I just need to spew it out. And then afterwards I can put my social worker brain back on and problem solve." And my supervisor was a hundred percent on board and knew where I was coming from and supportive of that. I just barged into her office that day and the whole time I was sad. But we've set the tone to where that's okay. After sharing my feelings she asked me, what are the steps moving forward? This question helps us as a staff so we do not get stuck griping about clients. We have freedom to express what's in our gut and then with support, we take a step

back and we think about the steps we want to take to move forward.

My supervisor has all of the components in her style of communicating with me that helps me to feel supported as a staff member. In our reflective supervision meetings—which we have about every two weeks—we begin with some task-oriented things. Checking in, how are things going, deadlines and stuff like that. Then I have a chance to share openly about issues I'm experiencing with families. **I'm able to vent without a filter.** Sometimes my own personal feelings get wrapped up in what's going on with the family and I feel safe to share those feelings. Then, we move on to the brainstorming and problem-solving phase. Before we end the meeting she always asks about my self-care: "What are you doing to take care of yourself? What can I do as a supervisor to support you?" She's been in the field, so she knows what we need and what we don't need. I also appreciate knowing that she is always available. I don't have to wait two weeks for our formal check-ins if there's something that is really pressing. She will always find time to be available for a conversation if I need one. And that really helps.

When I'm working with one of my colleagues who is really activated after an interaction with a family, I often draw on the practices we have learned through Touchpoints (www.brazeltontouchpoints.org/). One of the Touchpoints that always comes to mind is **value passion where you find it.** When a parent comes to us with a really abrasive approach, we try to stop and think, "well, where's this passion coming from?" They have a passion for something, whether that be the education of their child or the safety of their child or something else, there's a passion there. So if a colleague comes into the break room and they're processing their feelings with me about a family, I start by allowing them to vent and get their story and feelings out. I always acknowledge their frustration and how difficult the situation was for them.

And then, I might gently reframe the situation, using a strength-based approach, and encourage them to recognize the parent's passion. I might say, "it sounds like that parent is really passionate about X. I wonder if they're exhibiting this behavior because they feel really strongly about…."

The program Valendena works in understands the trauma-responsive principle, Understanding Stress and Trauma which we see being used by the supervisor in this vignette. Valendena's supervisor recognizes that when her staff are experiencing stress, managing uncertainty and feeling high emotions, they need a safe place to vent. Creating time and space for staff to let off "steam" in the presence of a trusted person who will listen without judgment and then guide them to identify strategies and actions they can take to move forward, is a trauma-responsive practice. The supervisor did not need to lecture, give advice, teach, redirect or say "calm down" because she knows that when we can release our built-up emotions, we will eventually calm and be able to access our cortex or "thinking and problem-solving brain." Valendena also describes a helpful example of using a strength-based approach in her work with families. When a parent or caregiver approaches her with intensity and what might be typically described as challenging or dysregulated behavior, she reframes it as passion and deep care for their child. Understanding that all behavior is communicating a story and knowing about the importance of looking underneath the behavior to explore what it is telling us about how parents feel and/or what they need, allows us to shift from a trauma-inducing approach (reactive) to a trauma-responsive approach (inviting curiosity, listening, seeking to understand) in our communication and interactions.

Reflection/Discussion Questions

♦ Do you have an example of a difficult interaction with a parent/family who approached you with intense emotions or even aggressive verbal interactions? What was the parent's behavior communicating to you? Were they trying to tell you about a worry or concern? Looking past the dysregulated behavior, were you able to see what they were passionate about?

◆ Do you have an example of a time when another colleague or parent/family came to you with a story attached to high levels of emotional intensity? Alternatively, do you have an example when someone did this for you?

- Were you able to listen without advising, directing, correcting or problem-solving?
- How did you use non-verbal strategies (body language, facial expressions) to convey that you were listening?
- How did you use your verbal strategies (acknowledging their words, tone of voice) to send a message that you were listening?
- Valendena used her supervisor to help her regulate. Who do you go to at work and/or outside of work to help you vent and then re-regulate when you are stressed?

In this final example, we see how Understanding Stress and Trauma is not only about acknowledging the trauma in children's and adults' lives but also, taking steps to promote healthy expression of those feelings so that they don't disrupt our ability to engage, to feel safe and to hijack us throughout the day. In this vignette we see how teacher Chantelle disrupts a child's ongoing distress by using a scripted story (see textbox below for definition) to help her to feel safe and to calm her nervous system.

' My daddy loves me. Just because he's not here, does not mean that he doesn't want to be with me."—Chantelle Marin, Lead Teacher, Educare, Omaha

We see a lot of trauma related to deportation. I had one little girl, Yeseny, whose father was deported and that was really hard to see. It was personal too because my husband's Hispanic and his father was deported as well. So I had a connection because I've seen how it affected him and the stories he shared about that. When Yeseny was struggling, I was able to make her a social story. The story started, "**My daddy loves me. Just because he's not here, does not mean that he doesn't want to be with me and he doesn't love me.**" I spoke with Yeseny's mom and asked her, "Can I have some pictures of dad? I think this would be nice for Yeseny to see pictures of her dad. We want to put them up in the classroom and make sure she knows he's there." Several of our families face similar situations. We have lots of families who are refugees. Several children have a mother or father incarcerated and we have children who are in the foster care system. We try to understand and acknowledge the trauma they have experienced but also work hard to create feelings of welcome and inclusion and to prevent them from feeling that their families are not respected or visible in our classrooms.

Mirrors, Windows and Sliding Glass Doors

Rudine Sims Bishop (1990) writes,

> Books are sometimes windows, offering views of worlds that may be real or imagined, familiar or strange. These windows are also sliding glass doors, and readers have only to walk through in imagination to become part of whatever world has been created or recreated by the author. When lighting conditions are just right, however, a window can also be a mirror. Literature transforms human experience and reflects it back to us, and in that reflection we can see our own lives and experiences as part of the larger human experience. Reading, then, becomes a means of self-affirmation, and readers often seek their mirrors in books...For many years, nonwhite readers have too frequently found the search futile.
>
> (p. 1)

Pastel et al. (2019) explain,

> All children need mirrors that reflect who they are and validate their existence, and all children need windows that validate the existence of others. But for many children—children of color and multiracial children, disabled children, children in non-nuclear family structures, neuro-atypical children, immigrant children, poor children, children of size and children in other marginalized cultural positions—too many books, stories told and cultural norms are *only* windows. They receive the message that they are inferior, not important enough to be reflected in literature, or worse, reflected only through negative stereotypes. For others—children in dominant cultural positions including White, able-bodied children from middle or upper class heterosexual nuclear families—too many books are *only* mirrors. These children receive the message that their experience is the norm.
>
> (p. 166)

Teacher Chantelle understood that one way to support Yeseny in the wake of her father's deportation was to help her feel his presence in the classroom: To ensure that he continued to be acknowledged as her father—a central attachment figure and family member in her life—despite his physical absence. By creating a scripted story that reflected back to Yeseny the story of the trauma of her father's deportation as well as the strengths, coping skills and supports that she and her mother had to help them continue on, Teacher Chantelle was acknowledging their trauma (creating a mirror for Yeseny's lived experience) while also highlighting their strengths and sources of resilience and reminders that they were not alone and had support from others to help them to cope and survive.

What are Scripted Stories?

Scripted Stories are written uniquely for an individual child who is having difficulty with a new life change, an expectation, facing a new situation, a new routine or that is having a hard time learning a social skill expectation. The story is written from the child's perspective and helps them identify how they feel and ways they can feel safe or follow the new routine or expectations.

https://carolgraysocialstories.com/social-stories/what-is-it/

http://csefel.vanderbilt.edu/scriptedstories/tips.pdf

www.pbisworld.com/tier-2/social-stories/

Working with children and families impacted by trauma will undoubtedly touch our own life experiences and may surface difficult feelings. As early childhood professionals, we can't help but be impacted through the stories of our families and children as they remind us of our own trauma, our own personal life story. Being trauma-responsive means cultivating self-awareness and self-care but also seeking support in times of emotional distress. There are many sources that can ground us in times of stress, so we don't allow our own stories and feelings that surface to adversely impact the children and families we work with. Supports may look like reflective supervision or intentional and culturally responsive self-care practices (Nicholson, Driscoll, Kurtz, Wesley & Benitez, 2020) that restore our stress or that help us feel grounded and safe. Sometimes people will need to seek additional mental health support when the issues become so overwhelming that they are adversely impacting their personal and/or professional life.

References

Bishop, R. S. (1990). Mirrors, windows, and sliding glass doors. Originally published in *Perspectives*, *1*(3), ix–xi. Retrieved from https://

scenicregional.org/wp-content/uploads/2017/08/Mirrors-Windows-and-Sliding-Glass-Doors.pdf.

Nicholson, J., Driscoll, P., Kurtz, J., Wesley, L. & Benitez, V. (2020). Culturally responsive self-care practices for early childhood educators. New York, NY: Routledge.

Pastel, E., Steele, K., Nicholson, J., Maurer, C., Hennock, J., Julian, J., Unger, T. & Flynn, N. (2019) *Supporting gender diversity in early childhood classrooms: A Practical Guide*. Shoals, IN: Kingsley Press.

Siegel, D., & Payne Bryson, T. (2015). *The whole brain child*. Eau Claire, WI: PESI Publishing and Media.

5

CORE PRINCIPLE: Acknowledge Systems of Privilege and Oppression and Take Actions to Disrupt Inequity

Learning to understand and critically examine the policies, practices and decisions that create stress and trauma and reproduce cycles of oppression—that harm parents and families in our programs, schools and systems—and taking actions that disrupt inequity, are important steps in building resilience and healing. Taking actions that avoid re-traumatization and disrupt the policies, practices and/ or conditions that harm children, families, communities and the workforce serving them provides individuals and groups with a sense of control, agency and purpose building blocks for strengthening resilience and supporting the healing process. Well-being comes from participating in transforming the underlying causes of harm within our societal structures and institutions (Ginwright, 2018).

Trauma-responsive family engagement in early childhood acknowledges the uneven playing field that exists for young

DOI: 10.4324/9781003127666-6

children and families and the early childhood workforce and emphasizes the importance of:

◆ Increasing awareness of what oppression is and how it is reproduced within early childhood organizations and systems leading many children and parents/families to be further harmed, marginalized and negatively impacted by trauma

◆ Increasing early childhood professionals' awareness of how they (personally) and the children and families they serve are positioned within systems of oppression and privilege and therefore, affected differently

◆ Guiding the early childhood field to take individual and collective actions to disrupt harm and inequity and to strengthen healing and wellness, especially for Black, indigenous and children and families of color

Increase Awareness About Oppression

Building a shared vocabulary to talk about oppression and privilege is an important first step for creating family engagement practices that disrupt harm and aim to be trauma responsive and healing centered.

What Is Oppression?

To oppress, is to "hold down—to press—and deny a social group full access to resources in a given society" (DiAngelo, 2016, p. 61). Oppression is what happens when one group—the **dominant** (or sometimes called the "agent" group) has the power to enforce their prejudice and discrimination against another group, the **minoritized** (or the "target" group) throughout the society (DiAngelo, 2016).

Examples of Different Forms of Oppression and Minoritized and Dominant Groups

Minoritized/Target group	Form of oppression	Dominant/Agent group
People of Color	Racism	White (or in some cases light skinned individuals)
Poor, working class	Classism	Middleclass, wealthy
People with disabilities	Ableism	Able-bodied
Elderly	Ageism	Young, middle-aged
Women	Sexism	Men

Source: Adapted from DiAngelo (2016, p. 64)

Oppression describes a process of prejudice and discrimination that is at a societal level (DiAngelo, 2016). How is a minoritized group "held down" by the dominant group? Through **policies, practices, traditions, norms, definitions, cultural stories, and explanations** (for events and/or circumstances) **that use a deficit perspective** to represent the minoritized group and give power and benefits solely to the dominant group (DiAngelo, 2016).

Prejudice + Discrimination + Power = Oppression

> Many of the existing frameworks of family engagement provide policy commitments or prescriptions that fail to address the complexities of how race, power, gender, language, class and other social markers shape family-school relations.
>
> (Ishimaru et al., 2019, p. 1)

For a more in-depth discussion of structural racism, the elements of oppression, understanding how we are positioned within systems of oppression and privilege and characteristics of dominant/White supremacy culture and antidotes for creating trauma-responsive healing centered early childhood environments see: Nicholson, J., Kurtz, J. Leland, J., Wesley, L., & Nadiv, S. (2021). *Trauma-Responsive Practices for Early Childhood Leaders: Creating and Sustaining Healing Engaged Organizations*. Routledge.

We don't do a good enough job in schools to acknowledge the harm that our schools perpetrate in communities of color and how just being part of the school system
in itself means that we are holding positions of power.
Even myself having grown up in a working-class immigrant family, and having grown up in an urban area
where I witnessed violence and experienced really hor-
rible things as a child, even being a survivor of abuse
myself, my experience is not the same as the families
right now, as the families of today, because I grew up in a
different context.

(Laura Rivas, Family Engagement Specialist,
Berkeley Unified School District)

Trauma-responsive family engagement acknowledges that we
must be willing to open conversations about the impact of privilege and oppression on parents and family members in early
childhood programs and services. What has been significantly
missing in language and frameworks addressing parent involvement and family engagement is an honest reckoning that early
childhood professionals cannot hope to build trust with families
who have been—and continue to be—silenced, marginalized,
positioned through deficit and harmed by the institutions and
systems that profess to support them (e.g., housing, child care,
health care, child welfare etc.).

Laura Rivas, a Family Engagement Specialist, in a large
urban school district provides an example in the vignette below
where she describes how racism impacts children and families
of color, especially Black families, on a daily basis within the
schools where she works.

**"Racial trauma is too often not acknowledged or discussed
but it significantly impacts our treatment of children and families"**—Laura Rivas, Family Engagement Specialist, Berkeley
Unified School District

The way that trauma has been spoken about in schools
feels like we put trauma on children of color. Like we see

children of color as traumatized. And so therefore, it's another stigma, another label just like "at risk youth" and I want to change that. Now we are talking about trauma-responsive family engagement which means that we would be responsive to *all of our trauma*. Every single one of us has trauma. It's a human experience. But it's also so important to acknowledge institutional systemic trauma. Too often, we focus only on the interpersonal trauma, "Oh, this child experienced abuse by their parent" which basically leads us to have a deficit mindset of a family and of the child, "They're traumatized." But we need to understand how trauma impacts children and families within a larger context. For example, racial trauma that people of color experience and the ways that this type of trauma manifests and leads us to put up walls or our collective inability to honestly engage in conversations around racial justice or racism. **Racial trauma is too often not acknowledged or discussed but it significantly impacts our treatment of children and families.** Given this, we need to consider what does trauma responsive mean? Because we can't leave ourselves out of it. We can't be like, "Oh, I'm going to be trauma responsive toward this student in this family, but I'm leaving myself completely out of it." If we're not willing to be changed or impacted ourselves, then we are not doing trauma-responsive work.

We also have to get rid of the scarcity mindset, "I can't care about everybody. I don't have enough love to go around." Actually, no, we do have enough love to go around and we must create room for everybody. We must include all of us. We can't be throwing people away and replicating the prison industrial complex in our schools and in our minds. "Oh this family, this poor child" we want to literally rescue the child from a family environment that we think is bad for them. But because of racial bias and the systems of oppression that live inside of us, we respond to children and families in ways that reflect racism and bias. For example, with a White family, we might be more compassionate and give them the benefit of the doubt. One clear way that I see this playing out in our district is with attendance. The way attendance is managed with White families whose children miss school and with children of color whose children miss school is a completely different process. White families are very rarely sent to truancy court for missing school. A White family could say, "We went to France for two weeks" and they would be believed, rarely asked to show their plane tickets and never be investigated. But if it's a Black family, well, I have accompanied more Black families in truancy court than any other racial group.

Before we can build trust with families impacted by oppression and structural racism, we must acknowledge and name the harms and trauma that have, and continue to, impact them and fuel their feelings of distrust with systems, programs, schools and services. Only by first acknowledging the roots and reasons underlying their distrust—e.g., the impact of bias and systems that perpetuate different outcomes for children and families based on race as reflected in Laura's story—and being willing to disrupt policies and practices that reproduce inequity, can we move forward in repairing harm and rebuilding the foundations of trust that are necessary for building positive relationships.

Before We Can Build Trust, We Must Acknowledge Histories and Sources of Distrust

Families and communities with histories of systemic and institutional mistreatment often develop distrust. Distrust arises when an individual or group does not believe that the decisions or actions made by others that impact their lives are reliable or based on a shared set of values or principles (Schultz, 2019). Another source of distrust results from hierarchical decision-making in which those with formal authority and in positions of power make decisions for people with less authority and power—when decisions are made *for* rather than *with* the community often ignoring their dreams or demands —therefore, reducing the amount of influence and agency/self-determination they have to control the decisions and factors that have significant impacts on their daily lives (Schultz, 2019). Moving from parent involvement to authentic power-sharing partnerships and family engagement will not succeed without acknowledging the historical distrust many parents and families—especially Black, Indigenous and Families of Color have with educational and social service systems, programs and services.

How do we as early childhood professionals begin the process of addressing distrust with parents and families? We must start with the courage and willingness to "uncover, acknowledge, honestly name, and directly address the genesis and sources of the distrust because without doing so, the solutions will be fleeting. The persistence of distrust can impede positive change and reform" (Schultz, 2019). Yet, honest dialogues that honestly name historical sources of distrust and oppression—e.g., racism, slavery, genocide, colonialism, disconnecting Indigenous Peoples from their "histories, landscapes, languages, social relations and their own ways of thinking, feeling and interacting with the world" (Thuiwai Smith, 2012, p. 29) are not yet happening across our society. It is therefore, understood why many historically marginalized families respond to invitations to participate and/or partner with early learning programs and services (especially those funded by the government) with fear, concern and caution. The trust of families and communities whose experiences of trauma and oppression have created a deep-seated sense of distrust will need to be earned. The injustices People of Color and Indigenous Peoples have faced in the U.S. span centuries and continue to the current day. As a result, the process of building trust will necessarily be long-term and contingent upon how effectively we individually and collectively address the root of the sources of distrust that exist.

Reflection/Discussion Questions

◆ When you read about the inequities created by institutional racism and oppression, what is your first reaction? Is this new to you? Familiar?

◆ Can you think of the ways you do or perhaps ways you could create opportunities for parents and families to share their lived experiences of inequity?

Acknowledging and Reducing Power Differentials in Communication and Interactions with Families

I ask a lot of questions and I do a lot of listening to parents and families. It's a huge investment of my time as a Family Engagement Specialist for our school district. I am aware that this is integral to my job and I can do this. I'm not expecting that every single teacher is able to do this to the same degree but there are certain things all teachers can do. Even in parent meetings or conferences, knowing that when parents are coming into a space with you, they are putting you up here and themselves down here, not everyone, but many of our parents of color are doing this. Understanding this dynamic in communication with families is essential for reducing the power differential.

(Laura Rivas, Family Engagement Specialist, Berkeley Unified School District)

An essential foundation of using a trauma-responsive approach in family engagement is understanding the role of power differentials and their ability to negatively impact people's feelings of safety and to trigger or activate their stress response systems. Bruce Perry (2020d) reminds us about the importance of appreciating and being aware of power differentials and how they play out in our daily interactions with others including parents and families. Without understanding and acknowledging these dynamics, our words, body language or actions can inadvertently communicate messages that cause others to feel unsafe or even threatened. When this happens—we may struggle to understand why our words, invitations to connect and to partner are being met with indifference, resistance, anger, frustration or behavior that is surprising and/or confusing.

Dr. Perry (2020d) describes how and why power differentials are present in our interactions with others:

> ...In our brain, we have this neurobiological set of systems designed to continually monitor the social milieu. To basically get a sense of how safe we are. Do we belong? Your brain is literally nonstop doing this social monitoring to get a sense of where you fit into the group...Our stress response systems are tremendously influenced by our sense of whether or not we belong to the group or if we're getting signals that we don't belong....Somebody who is given signals of acceptance, they feel safe. They feel like they belong...they are literally getting this bath of powerful, physiological regulation and reward and opportunities to have a fully open cortex so that they can learn things on an ongoing basis...When we are in the presence of people that we don't know, or people who are not sending us signals of inclusion and acceptance, it activates our stress response. It makes us feel threatened. If you start to feel like you don't quite belong, this is something that is really important because it begins to influence how we are functioning cognitively, how we are functioning behaviorally, how we are feeling emotionally and how our physiology is managing our stress response...the more threatened we feel, the more the lower parts of our brains start to dominate and control our functioning. And sometimes we're not even consciously aware of the threat. It impacts our physiology, and we may feel uncomfortable, but we're not really appreciating the degree to which it influences the way we think and feel. This is what creates the power differential.

Given our neurobiology and the way our brains are wired, it is important that early childhood professionals understand that just being in a position of power (e.g., teacher versus parent/ family member, home visitor versus family member, Family Engagement Specialist versus parent) can be triggering for a parent or family member we are interacting with. The less safe or welcome they feel in our presence or in the early learning program, school or agency, and the more they perceive that they are in a subdominant position within the power differential (Perry, 2020d), the more likely they are to display stress-related behaviors. And when they perceive that they are in situations where they have little power and control (e.g., a parent conference) the more likely you are to see stress-related behaviors like shutting down, compliance, disengagement, short comments or a lack of responsiveness. What does this look like? A parent drops their child off at the preschool program and the teacher mentions when she is signing out, "Can we talk soon? I have a few things I have been observing that I want to talk to you about." The parent responds, "I am so sorry, but I have to rush out to another commitment I have…maybe next time." The next few weeks, the teacher observes the parent on the phone every time at drop off and pick up. This is an example of a parent moving into that stressed or freeze state to protect themselves from the perceived danger they feel after this request to meet from the teacher.

> When you have one person interacting with another person, both of their brains are using this very important, very powerful neurobiology of connectedness. Part of what happens is **there is an automatic power differential that gets set up between individuals**…if you meet with a peer and you feel safe and comfortable with them, there's not a lot of difference between you and them with regards to this power differential, but there are all kinds of things that will in interactions with others, create a differential between the most dominant and the subdominant person. And that creates a power differential. The bigger, the power differential, and the more threatened you feel, the more the lower parts of your brain start to dominate and control your function. So, if you felt safe and comfortable, you are able to be driven and controlled by the

smartest part of your brain (cortex). But when there's a huge power differential, people get pushed down the arousal continuum. One of the most common behaviors of somebody who's in a subdominant position with a dominant person is that they are behaviorally frozen... (e.g., compliant, robotic responses with few words spoken)... if you're not aware of the way in which your status or your dominance puts people at a cognitive disadvantage, you're going to have a hard time communicating.

(Perry, 2020d)

Just being in an educational setting or speaking to a teacher/provider/home visitor/mental health consultant/family engagement specialist/supervisor can be triggering for some adults, reminding them of their own past experiences in school or working within systems where they had traumatic experiences they associate with feelings of a total loss of control, powerlessness and fear. There are many examples we could think of including a lack of safety due to racism, class discrimination, being defined through deficit, lack of cultural or linguistic alignment in the school, fear due to their undocumented status, being expelled, witnessing a school shooting and many others.

Working with a trauma-responsive approach requires that we understand, acknowledge and work to increase safety and decrease power differentials in our interactions with parents and families. When someone is at the bottom of the power differential, they will behave and act in ways that are a response to a perceived threat (being in a subdominant position; see Chapter 2 on state-dependent functioning). If we do not understand how our words or actions can lead parents and families to feel threatened and perceive they are at the more vulnerable end of a power hierarchy, we may find their responses to our communication, invitations, directions or requests for information to be confusing and/or frustrating if their behavior reflects a stress-related reaction to a perceived threat.

As early childhood professionals, we want to be continually aware of our positionality and consider, how can I even the playing field? How can I decrease my power and communicate messages of safety, inclusiveness and respect to parents and families? We need to think about this whenever we enter a child's home, when we lead a meeting with a family and in the many interactions we have throughout our daily work with parents and family members.

What Can Early Educators Do to "Even the Playing Field" and Decrease the Power Differential during Our Interactions with Parents and Families?

Given the realities of our neurobiology that leads our brains to automatically create power differentials in our relationships and interactions with others, what can we do to reduce this effect? What can we do to decrease parents' and families' perceptions of threat and sub-dominance when we are interacting with them? It turns out that there is a lot we can do to intentionally communicate messages that decrease threat and instead, reinforce feelings of safety, respect and partnership. It is essential that early educators understand what factors minimize the power differential and what they can do to decrease its impact in our engagement with families. For example:

◆ Start with a humanizing mindset. Recognize that early childhood professionals *and* parents and families all have valuable expertise and one partner is not more important or valuable than the other.

Mother Teresa has always been one of my heroes. She said that there is not one single person on the face of the earth who is more important than another person. We all just have different responsibilities. And that's what I want for our school. There is not one single person who is more important than the next. That is a way to think about and help families when they're experiencing stress. They have such huge reasons to be stressed, but I think if you have a foundation and an expectation that every parent, every family matters, they are all respected in this place, that's huge.

(Kristina Adams, Program Director, Hayward Unified School District Early Learning Program)

When we actively view all families as bringing strengths and assets to our program and we communicate messages as Kristina does that *"nobody in this program is more important than any other person"*—we are shifting mindsets to see parents as equal partners which will increase the likelihood that we can build trust and positive relationships with them and begin to disrupt power imbalances. However, when one partner has perceived power "over" the other (i.e., a supervisor who can determine whether a parent receives services or a mental health consultant conducting home visits), then we automatically reinforce the power differential. Families perceive this imbalance every day whether it is stated or not. There are many steps we can take to disrupt the power differential so that families feel safe, welcome and have an inherent belief that their voice matters. Kristina Adams describes a simple but profound way she does this with the parents and families in her program: by starting with a philosophy and taking small acts in her everyday interactions to help families believe that her door is always open and that they matter to her, their voice and presence matters. **As Bettina Love (2019) reminds us, "mattering" is essential** for individuals and groups that have historically been marginalized.

◆ Learn about and acknowledge the existence of power imbalances and commit to being intentional in taking actions to reduce them

It is essential to appreciate and build awareness of the power differential—and the way our beliefs and behaviors contribute to messages of dominance and sub-dominance—in our moment-to-moment communication and interactions with parents and families. We can communicate to families that they have essential importance and valued expertise in our partnership and that who they are and what they bring to the relationship matters. Valentina Torres, a marriage and family therapist who conducts home visits with many newly arrived refugee and immigrant families describes below how she assumes this mindset in her work.

"I intentionally work to level the playing field"—Valentina Torres, Early Childhood Mental Health Specialist, Jewish Family and Children's Services

> In my work with immigrant families, I find that there is a tendency to defer to power. And in my work with them, I come into the relationship in a position of power. And so there's a reverence that they automatically give me that I immediately appreciate but also, at the same time, **I intentionally work to level the playing field.** What does that mean? I reassure them that I'm coming in and I have some knowledge in some areas, but they too have important knowledge in others. This is a really important first step being trauma responsive in family engagement. I really try to highlight some strengths of families. There is an initial tendency to see me as someone coming in from the government and that I represent power and hierarchy and what I see is that they really shut down in front of me. And so, building rapport with them is important so that they understand that yes, I do come from the system and I need to monitor and call CPS and do all these things to ensure the safety of young children, but I can also hold their truths and I will treat them respectfully as an equal. I do not ever think I'm better than anyone else. I just have a different skill set and different kinds of knowledge. Taking this approach is what helps me to build rapport with families as I want them to understand how much I care about whatever situation they're in and that whatever happened to them, whether it was against their will or because of their own judgment and by their own hand, there's value in who they are and that things can get better.

Valentina knows that when she enters the home of a family she is automatically in a position of power. She is aware of this power and the impact it has on families, the stress it may cause them, the trauma it may trigger. She intentionally takes steps and actions to "even the power differential" so that families see her as human and feel safe with her. This can take time. But we must have awareness as the first step and take action to help families feel valued, seen and to decrease the power differential.

Jenje, a toddler teacher and home visitor in Los Angeles, has a similar practice. Whenever she enters a family home, she reinforces her position as a "learner" to communicate that she may have expertise in some areas but in others she is very much learning just like the families. In the following example she explains how she positions the families as experts in speaking Spanish and learners of English and for her it is the reverse:

> When I enter the homes of our families, I try to speak to them in Spanish. When the families tell me "we don't speak English well," I respond, "¡No, te preocupes!" They laugh and I laugh and I reassure them that I am trying to learn the Spanish language too just like you are learning English. This helps to break the barriers down and helps us to connect. It helps me set the tone that I am not coming into their homes to judge them. I'm a Black person with dreadlocks walking into your Latinx home learning Spanish just as you are learning to speak English.
> (Jenje Dennis, toddler teacher and home visitor)

◆   Center the voices of parents and families in decision-making

We can address the roots of distrust and work towards building power-sharing partnerships with parents and families by centering *their* voices in the development of the policies, procedures and practices that guide our early childhood programs and services. Centering parents and families and inviting them to influence our early childhood programs and services with their ideas and stories, creates an opportunity for emergent listening. When we truly listen to what they tell us, we have an opportunity to *disrupt our listening as usual* and to be open to new possibilities and to **being affected and willing to change in response to what we hear families say.** One elementary school that centered the families' voices in a discussion of early elementary curriculum expanded the topics they were considering after learning from parents that addressing bullying and fostering children's positive racial identities were both important topics they wanted addressed in the curriculum that neither the teachers or administrators were considering:

> Centering nondominant parent perspectives meant **beginning from their priorities** to decide the curriculum topics, some atypical to previous programming by the school. For example their ongoing experiences with bullying and shared history of frustration surrounding their efforts to address it with educators created an important parent curriculum topic for their communities. In addition, [the] parents also introduced "Fostering Positive Racial Identity" to the educators as an important element for improving student outcomes...one of the teachers on the team described her profound learning about the importance of racial identity in student learning and subsequently taught other teachers about racial microaggressions in the classroom, crediting the parents with building her understanding of those dynamics... Without centering parent priorities as part of the collaboration process, it is likely that these topics may not have made the final cut as many educators did not see these topics as central.
>
> (Ishimaru et al., 2019)

By centering families' voices—especially those least likely to be heard—and allowing them to truly influence our policies and practices we will learn from their knowledge, experiences and expertise as true partners. Centering families' voices can be an important part of the process of communicating respect to families and disrupting the inequities so many have experienced and continue to experience in systems, programs and schools that do not honor the strengths, knowledge and wisdom they bring into the relationship and process of educating their children.

Dr. Bruce Perry (2020d) recommends several additional ways we can use to reduce power differentials in our relationships and interactions including with parents and families:

- ◆ **Understand that simply having repeated contact/ interactions with people can lead to reduced perceptions of threat**. The more frequently we see someone and have even brief moments of relational connection with them, the less our brains will perceive threat in their presence. Therefore, simply having repetitive contact with parents and family members reduces uncertainty and increases familiarity which can improve their unconscious perceptions of safety in our presence.

- ◆ **Be intentional about the verbal and non-verbal signals you send in your communication.** Build awareness of your facial expressions, tone of voice and the questions you ask when you communicate with parents and families. Do your best to avoid sending any abrupt cues and be intentional about sending verbal and non-verbal messages of reassurance and support (e.g., asking for consent and giving them choices—"Is now a good time to talk? I would love to learn from you about…," smile, use a calm tone of voice and use warm and welcoming body language like open versus folded arms). Learn which formats of communication are most accessible and preferred by different families (e.g., text messaging might be most effective for some families while others prefer face-to-face conversations).

- ◆ **Understand how physical size, physical proximity and gaze impact feelings of threat and safety**. Physical size and proximity can be important factors in a power differential. If you are interacting with someone who is much larger than you or if someone stands close and this is someone we don't know or do not trust, this move can be perceived as an expression of dominance and it can trigger a stress reaction, especially for someone larger than us. It is important to be mindful of your size (in comparison to a parent or family member), your physical proximity during interactions with parents and families and to try to avoid making quick movements towards someone as this could decrease their sense of felt safety. Additionally, it is helpful to prevent a situation where families have to look up to you during a conversation. Putting them in a position where they have to use an upward gaze to communicate with you could automatically activate their brain's survival response as this would signal that they are in the subdominant position within the relationship (e.g., try to avoid having them sit on a couch or in a chair that is lower than you). The following two examples reflect early childhood professionals who are aware of these factors and intentionally try to reduce the power hierarchy in their work with families:

A home visitor enters the home, and the family sits on the chairs and couch in the living room. She asks, "Is there a place you would like me to sit?" The family says anywhere you like to and she then asks them, "Is it okay if I sit on the floor with your child and play with him while we meet?" She intentionally signals to the parents that she is willing to sit lower than they do (so she would have an upper gaze to them during the conversation) but she also gives them agency and control to decide where she sits.

A parent/teacher conference meeting is scheduled and when the parent arrives, the teacher provides a warm welcome and invitation for tea or water. The teacher invites the parent to choose which seat feels most comfortable for them first and then, the teacher offers paper and pen to the parent to take notes or to doodle so that they don't have to have sustained eye contact. The teacher is creating a safe and predictable environment and reducing any perceived threat by centering the parent's voice and their needs from the moment they enter the meeting space. She helps the parent to feel safe by providing small opportunities to regulate (paper to doodle or take notes) and by creating a warm welcome (offering a drink, providing a choice for seating). The teacher is acutely aware that a meeting like this can trigger emotions and a feeling of powerlessness for a family and that creating safety for them is essential.

◆ **Create opportunities for parents and families to have "voice and choice."** When parents and families perceive that they have no choice and no voice they are more likely to be triggered into a fight, flight or freeze stress response. The antidote to this is creating opportunities for families to have agency and control in their interactions and in early childhood environments. Specific strategies and ideas for increasing families' agency and control are introduced and discussed throughout Chapter 6.

◆ **Build awareness of diverse cultural beliefs and unconscious bias that impact perceptions of power**. Culture has a profound influence on our perceptions of power— what we assume is natural, normal and/or desired in terms of the way power dynamics play out among individuals of different genders, races, abilities, roles, ages, etc. Similarly, we all have unconscious biases that significantly impact how we perceive the world and our place within it. These biases have a significant influence on how we perceive safety, inclusion/exclusion and threat. Building awareness of cultural differences and the impact unconscious bias has in our relationships and interactions with parents and families is an important part of learning how and why power differentials develop and the actions we can take in different contexts to reduce parents' and families' perceptions of our "power over" them.

Reflection/Discussion Questions

◆ How do you or your program build trust with families? What specific strategies do you use to slowly build trust over time?

- When engaging with families at school, in their home or by phone, what strategies do you use to "even the playing field" or reduce the real or perceived "power differential" as Valentina does?
- Can you think of an example when you took the stance of "learner" like Jenje to communicate with a family that you are thinking partners together?
- In what ways do you create intentional opportunities for families to provide input into program development, policies or to co-construct curriculum?

References

DiAngelo, R. (2016). *What does it mean to be White? Developing White racial literacy* (Revised ed.). New York, NY: Peter Lang.

Ginwright, S. (2018). *The future of healing: Shifting from trauma informed care to healing centered engagement*. Medium.

Ishimaru, A., Lott, J., Torres, K. & O-Reilly-Diaz, K. (2019). Families in the driver's seat: Catalyzing familial transformative agency for equitable collaboration, *Teachers College Record*, *121*(11), 1–39. www.tcrecord.org ID Number: 22819.

Love, B. (2019). *We want to do more than survive: Abolitionist teaching and the pursuit of educational freedom*. Boston, MA: Beacon Press.

Nicholson, J., Kurtz, J., Leland, J., Wesley, L. & Nadiv, S. (2021). *Trauma-responsive practices for early childhood leaders: Creating and sustaining healing engaged organizations*. New York: Routledge.

Ferry, B. (2020d). Understanding the power differential. NN COVID Series 12. Retrieved from https://youtu.be/ulwfwYDffV8.

Schultz, K. (2019). *Distrust and educational change: Overcoming barriers to just and lasting reform*. New York, NY: Teachers College Press.

Tuiwai Smith, L. (1999/2012). *Decolonizing methodologies: Research and indigenous peoples* (2nd ed.). London: Zed Books.

6

CORE PRINCIPLE: Establish Safety and Predictability

Trauma impacts parents' and families' perceptions of safety. Establishing physical, social and emotional safety, and reducing uncertainty (by increasing regularity and predictability in relationships and environments) increases individuals' feelings of safety and belonging. Parents' and families' stress is reduced in relationships and within environments that communicate feelings of safety, calm and predictability.

> As soon as a family walks in, the first thing we need to make sure is that we smile with them and we say, "hello." We acknowledge them with a welcoming face.
> (Rosalee Estrada, Family Engagement Specialist)

Establishing safety and predictability is perhaps the most critical need in a trauma-responsive approach to family engagement. As described previously, parents' past and current experiences of oppression, marginalization and/or trauma in their lives and simply the wide range of stressors many encounter on a daily basis can make this responsibility quite challenging. When

DOI: 10.4324/9781003127666-7

people experience trauma, their stress response systems can be rewired to be on "high alert" and continually tell them that they are unsafe. This can disrupt their ability to read cues accurately in others and within the environment and may alter their amygdala (brain alarm system) to be set off more than usual. This is why it is so important for early childhood professionals to learn how to help children, parents and families to feel safe in our everyday interactions and in the environment they enter and in the words we use.

The number one trauma-responsive strategy to rewire the activated stress response systems is nurturing, responsive relationships and safe, predictable environments. As we read the vignette below, can you identify how Child Development Resources established a sense of safety and predictability when faced with a community crisis?

"We paused to make sure that our staff and our families were okay."—Aracely Nava, Family Engagement Coordinator, Child Development Resources, Ventura

> Our community experienced many natural disasters this year that have impacted our staff and the families that we serve including the big Thomas fire that devastated our county. A lot of people had to leave their homes and many lost their jobs. Many of our staff couldn't work for a while as they had to evacuate their homes. What our management did, which I thought was extremely trauma informed, is **they paused to make sure that our staff and our families were okay**. Our centers were closed temporarily. Management wanted to make sure that the staff were taken care of so first and foremost, they checked in with all of us to see what we needed. They reinforced that we could time off as we needed because of everything that was going on. For me, it was important that we paused; we didn't just keep going as a program. It's true that we have contractual requirements we always have to meet, but during this time, it was even more important that there was a recognition of what we, as a staff, needed

and our agency, we literally paused. They made sure that we were okay. After the staff were taken care of, we came together and we supported the families. It was a whole trauma-responsive and comprehensive approach. We collected donations for our families including diapers, water and baby things. We partnered with our local mental health agency and we offered crisis intervention groups for families and staff who were impacted by the fires. We also supported our children. We created opportunities for children to have a space to be able to talk about the fire in a developmentally appropriate manner with clinicians. And parents had support to learn how they could talk to their children about the fire. And so we addressed our community trauma from top to bottom using what was, for me, a very trauma informed approach.

> The Thomas fire was a massive wildfire that burned in 2017 in Southern California for two months over approximately 400 square miles, destroying over 1,000 structures, causing over $2.2 billion in damages and forcing over 104,000 residents to evacuate. It is currently the fifth-largest wildfire in the history of the state. Aracely's program, Child Development Resources (CDR) was located at the epicenter of the 2017 Thomas Fire and their community was devastated as staff and families faced trauma, loss and threats to their health and safety.

Aracely's agency understands that trauma (past or present) can impact people's perceptions of safety and that establishing physical, social and emotional safety is central to trauma-responsive resilience building environments in times of adversity. The agency staff were able to reduce stress because of several trauma-responsive actions their leadership took including:

◆ Pausing instead of reacting
◆ Encouraging the staff to take care of their needs first so they could then show up for families in an attuned and calming manner

- ◆ Acknowledging peoples' stress and addressing their basic needs
- ◆ Creating environments that reinforced a sense of welcome, safety and predictability
- ◆ Using the strength and resilience of the group to model and build resilience together by taking actions to address their individual and collective stressors and worries

Reflection/Discussion Questions

- ◆ In your work with parents/families, do you have an example of when you promoted the trauma-responsive principle of Safety and Predictability during a time of uncertainty, stress and/or during a traumatic event?
- ◆ In your example above were you able to take similar steps such as those implemented by Aracely's agency:
    - Pausing instead of reacting?
    - Filling your cup/taking care of your needs first so you can show up for families in an attuned and calming manner?
    - Acknowledging peoples' stress and addressing their needs?
    - Creating an environment that reinforces welcome, safety and predictability?
    - Using the strength and resilience of the group to model and build resilience by taking actions to address peoples' stressors and worries?

In the next vignette, Laura Rivas, Family Engagement Specialist, explains that creating a sense of safety and predictability for families is hard work and that their feelings of safety and trust are earned over time. Relationships take time to build and we must individualize our strategies for each family.

"Any interaction has to include listening and learning from both sides. We have to really be willing to humanize each other"—Laura Rivas, Family Engagement Specialist, Berkeley Unified School District

I work with two principals who are amazing Latina women who also grew up in working-class immigrant families like I did. Sometimes I feel like we fall into making the assumption that because we have a similar upbringing, that somehow that will translate into instant trust. But in reality, it still takes work. Our own lived experiences and identities matter, but they don't give us a free pass from doing the work of getting to know a family and their own unique lived experience. In true family engagement, nothing's automatic. It's really about doing the work to earn peoples' trust, being in a position with access to institutional power and being willing to share that power with a family. What I often tell families is I want to be your access point in the school. Inside the school, if you need me to be your voice, I can do that. Or, if you just need support to use your own voice, that would be my ideal. You already have a voice. I might know some things from working in the system that could be helpful to you. Oftentimes I have sat with families who want to speak with their child's teacher, but don't always know what to say, how to ask the questions or how to respond if the teacher says "no" to their requests. So I might suggest, "You could try this approach" and it's kind of like coaching our families not to give up and to advocate for their children in ways that are effective. But also to create a safe place in their child's school, where they can just be—free from judgment—with all of their feelings and deep vulnerability and powerlessness which often appears as defensiveness or avoidance/shut down.

Creating safe environments requires that early childhood professionals acknowledge the experiences that families have had with racism and bias in our schools and programs on a regular basis and how this impacts their feelings (or lack thereof) of safety, their ability to trust and/or to engage. As you read the vignette below, can you recognize how unconscious bias based on past experiences can be carried over to future interactions and disrupt our ability to create predictability and safety for families?

My approach with teachers is similar because for teachers, it can be very scary to be vulnerable with a family, especially when they have had negative experiences working with families. Like, "There was this one parent two years ago that yelled at me" and similar things that teachers carry with them. And if that parent happened to be African American, Latinx, Chinese or another specific background, then the next time they are confronted with a parent of that race, ethnicity or background, because of the way our brains make associations and our implicit biases, just seeing that person could create certain visceral reactions—triggers—in their body. And if they are not aware of that, it can impact how they talk to parents, how they listen to families, how they interpret others' behaviors. Many times teachers find themselves in conflictual situations with families and they don't understand how they got there. How did we end up with such different perspectives? How did this parent end up getting so angry and filing a complaint? When we trace back and reflect on all the small interactions, it's usually really clear the points where there were small microaggressions or violations of trust or not truly seeing the parent as an equal. So as educators, it's really important to have solid tools under our belt and a different mindset and approach when working with families who have been historically and systemically marginalized within schools and educational institutions (and sometimes the teachers too). Trust and relationship building are key in family engagement and they both take work, the kind of work one can only do when our commitment goes beyond our role as teacher or educator and we understand that our journeys are bound together. In one of the schools where I work, we have adopted the Mayan philosophy of In Lak 'Ech, meaning that we are all interconnected. The entire community of staff, students and families recite this beautiful poem every Friday morning:

In Lak 'Ech
You are my other me

> If I do harm to you, I do harm to myself
> If I love and respect you, I love and respect myself
> (Poem by Luis Valdez)

We will not be successful in supporting families to feel a sense of safety in our early learning programs unless we also acknowledge the sources of distrust. Laura acknowledges in the vignette above that we need to build awareness that many families experience microaggressions, racism and bias in our schools and programs and this impacts their own felt sense of safety. But when we enter into any interaction, we don't know exactly what a family has been through or how they feel. So, we have to engage in ways that seek to promote safety and recognize that when reactions come at us that we don't understand, we can take steps to make repairs, not react and definitely not abandon them.

What Are Racial Microaggressions and How Do They Show Up in our Work?

Microaggressions are brief and commonplace daily verbal, behavioral, or environmental actions (whether intentional or unintentional) that communicate hostile, derogatory, or negative racial slights and insults toward members of oppressed or targeted groups including: People of Color, women, Lesbian, Gay, Bisexual and Transgender (LGBT) persons, persons with disabilities, and religious minorities. Some scholars today argue that racism, sexism, homophobia, and other forms of discrimination are no longer as blatant as they may have been in the past. Instead, people may demonstrate their biases and prejudices in more subtle ways, otherwise known as microaggressions.

(Nadal, 2014, p. 71)

Derald Wing Sue and colleagues (2007) distinguish three types of microaggressions:

Microassaults—intentional acts of racism designed to harm a Person of Color (e.g., a wait staff member giving preferential treatment to a White person over a Person of Color, using racist language)

Microinsults—possibly unintentional acts of racism that deliver a hidden message insulting to a Person of Color (e.g., statements that imply People of Color received a job or promotion based on their skin color)

Microinvalidations—Messages that diminish the lived realities of People of Color (e.g., being asked, "Why do you always have to make things about race?" or being told, "I don't see race. I'm color blind" (Singh, 2019, pp. 105–106)).

The first step to addressing/disrupting racial micro-aggressions is to notice when they occur. The following table provides several examples (Source: Singh, 2019, p. 107).

Themes	Racial microaggression	Message
Alien in own land When Asian Americans and Latinx Americans are assumed to be foreign born	"Where are you from?" "Where were you born" "You speak good English."	You are not American.
	A person asking an Asian American to teach them words in their native language.	You are a foreigner.
Ascriptions of intelligence Assigning intelligence to a Person of Color based on their race	"You are a credit to your race."	People of Color are usually not as intelligent as Whites.
	"You are so articulate."	It is unusual for someone of your race to be intelligent.
	Asking an Asian person to help with math.	All Asians are intelligent and good in math/sciences.
Second-class citizen Occurs when a White person is given preferential treatment as a consumer over a Person of Color	Person of Color mistaken as a service worker	People of Color are servants to Whites. They couldn't possibly occupy high-status positions.
	Having a taxi cab pass a Person of Color and pick up a White passenger	You are likely to cause trouble and/or travel to a dangerous neighborhood.

Themes	Racial microaggression	Message
	Being ignored at a store counter as attention is given to the White customer behind you.	Whites are more valued customers than People of Color. You don't belong. You are a lesser being.
Color blindness Statements that indicate a White person does not want to acknowledge race	"When I look at you, I don't see color."	I am denying your racial/ethnic experiences as a Person of Color.
	"America is a melting pot."	Assimilate/acculturate to the dominant culture. I am denying you as a racial/cultural being.
	"There is only one race, the American race."	

Reflection/Discussion Questions

Identify the themes, microaggressions and messages in the following scenarios:

◆ Marta, who moved to the United States from El Salvador 15 years ago was in a staff meeting and asked to share a little bit about herself. When she mentioned where she was from, one colleague responded, "Wow, your English is so good."

◆ "Wow! You are so articulate! 'You're so well spoken.' Someone expressing shock or surprise by the fact that as a Black woman I speak using grammatically correct sentences sending a clear message that this was not their expectation and being smart is unusual"

◆ I was once volunteering at a private school, assisting with childcare for a faculty Back to School night. At the end of the evening, an older White administrator approached me and said, "¿Dónde está la basura?" (Where is the trash can?) and handed me her trash (which I did not take). Before I could respond, she repeated her question to me again in Spanish. Although I fully understood what she was saying, I was floored because I am not of Latinx descent. In fact, I am a non-Spanish speaking Black woman. Additionally, I was not the custodial staff, so the fact that she ascribed a profession along with my ethnicity was offensive.

♦ What type of response would you have had if you were misidentified as the person in the third scenario?
♦ What do you think a person who experiences a racial microaggression might be feeling or need?
♦ What response might you consider verbalizing to a person who commits a microaggression?[1]
♦ Are you able to recall an instance when you expressed a microaggression? If not, why do you think that is?
♦ What is our collective and individual responsibility to commit to equity, social justice and inclusion? How does learning about microaggressions support this?

When we think about creating safety in environments, our focus cannot be limited to the parents and families as early childhood professionals of color, including Family Engagement specialists like Laura, endure the same cycles and consequences of oppression that families experience. Having their voices and professional expertise invisibilized/marginalized and being the target of racial microaggressions from White families and colleagues prevents a program from becoming trauma-responsive. Safety can only be created in environments where individuals feel seen, heard and respected and where there is an honest acknowledgment of racism, concrete steps toward repairing harm (aka accountability), and ongoing anti-racist actions and reflections taken. Laura describes some of the barriers that get in the way of implementing trauma-responsive family engagement:

What gets in the way of implementing equity-committed family engagement practices? Well, a lot. To start with, one of the schools where I work is staffed with about 70% White teachers and the student population is 60% students of color. Working with this staff has been really difficult for me. I've had to reflect a lot on my own barriers to using my voice and just taking up space as a classified staff member who doesn't have a teaching credential. There's definitely a hierarchy in public education. If you don't have a teaching credential, it's almost like your expertise doesn't matter. Teachers are not going to listen to you unless you have an administrative or a teaching credential. It's unfortunate because so many of us who are classified staff (majority People of Color) have a wealth of knowledge to offer in how we relate with students and families of color.

It has taken years for some teachers, particularly White teachers and more veteran teachers, to see me as an expert and to just respond to their requests/demands for my support. "This family is hard to reach. Can you help me get them to do what I'm asking them to do?" It's been really hard to get the teachers to really listen to the feedback I offer. And then I think to myself, "If it's this hard to get them to listen to a colleague, how do they listen to families?" And so I am left to process all of these experiences on my own. I have to process all the little microaggressions from my White colleagues as a woman of color working with a majority White staff.

This story illustrates the importance of White staff having affinity groups and other spaces (reflection groups for White staff) to learn about privilege and racism without making this the responsibility of our colleagues of color. As we read on to the example below, we will learn of the hope and transformation that is possible when Black, Indigenous, People of Color and White colleagues build enough trust to have honest conversations about the beliefs, language and behaviors that reduce or eliminate feelings of safety for adults and children in minoritized groups. And then based on what is revealed, to have restorative conversations, to "listen and learn from both sides" and to "humanize each other" in moving forward.

> I've been proud of myself that I've been able to push through with some colleagues who have been open to reflecting, learning, and growing. We've had some big breakthroughs. One teacher, Mrs. Conley, and I have really different personalities. She's just someone who is going, going, going all the time and she would talk over me and I wouldn't get a chance to say anything. She was having a really difficult time with an African American family and it escalated pretty badly. I had warned her about her approach and suggested, "You might try something else. Something makes me uncomfortable about the way you treated this child and the way you spoke to the parent, this text, I wouldn't communicate this message via text." The conflict got worse and the teacher was distraught because she couldn't believe that the parent was so irate that he yelled at her in front of other children. It was terrible. In no way would I ever justify or defend that particular parent's behavior. But, the teacher and I had a really hard conversation about racial bias and the teacher was really willing to reflect, which was important. There were some things that I said that landed really harshly and she came back the next day, armed with courage to be vulnerable, and told me honestly how she felt. I had to be willing to listen to her with an open heart and without getting defensive and said, "You know what, you're right. I could have said that in a different way. Maybe it wasn't the right time as it was too fresh. I can recognize that." So we had to have that type of healing and restorative conversation. **Any interaction has to include listening and learning from both sides. We have to really be willing**

to humanize each other and approach each other with as much grace as we can. None of these are easy jobs. Parenting and teaching are two of the hardest jobs on this planet. I've seen what can happen when both parties are willing to work on building trust together. In my experience, building trust and creating safety with families requires that teachers develop dispositions for engaging in deep self-reflection and learning about anti-racism and for White teachers, it also involves recognizing their own privilege.

Mrs. Conley was working on understanding privilege and racism and making changes in her teaching. In this particular situation which reflected prejudiced beliefs and biases related to anti-Blackness, we went really deep in talking about it together. Now, she will come to me before speaking with the family and ask, "What do you think about this? I wasn't sure so I wanted to check with you." So we have that type of trust now. I don't think any less of her for seeking support or feedback. I think that's incredible and takes a lot of courage to be that vulnerable as an experienced teacher. We should be able to do this type of learning without fear of judgment or feeling like you failed. Oftentimes there's so much fear, "Oh, that one family, I just really messed up." Many teachers have shared with me that there are things that haunt them.—Laura Rivas, Family Engagement Specialist

In our interactions with others, there will always be difficult conversations and interactions. A sign of a healthy relationship is not one absent of conflict. It is how we have the hard conversations, how we make repairs, how we listen and engage that becomes trauma-responsive and healing engaged. Safety and Predictability is a core trauma-responsive principle highlighted in the vignette we just read. We see that creating safety happens by listening to others even if we feel different. Safety happens when we take a stance of humility and convey a message that there is room for more than one idea, viewpoint and opinion other than mine. When we listen— especially with an openness to being changed by what we hear, we create safety. But the vignette goes beyond safety to reflect other trauma-responsive principles—Creating Power Sharing Partnerships where we honor all the voices that are in the room and Acknowledging Systems of Privilege and Oppression and Taking Actions to Disrupt Inequity as seen in the relationship Laura built with her colleague Mrs. Conley that led to both of them humanizing one another and Mrs. Conley taking steps to acknowledge and then disrupt her language and actions based on racial bias.

Reflection/Discussion Questions

♦ When having a difficult interaction or conversation, in what ways do you create safety and predictability by addressing inequity and/or creating power sharing partnerships? Specifically, by listening, making sure there is space for others' voices and by not just listening with your ears but also acknowledging how they feel, their intention and the strengths of what they are bringing and conveying?

CORE PRINCIPLE: Acknowledge Strengths and Assets

For me, the major shift in the 28 years of doing work in family engagement, has been moving from a deficit-based view—"Parents are in need," "Families need to learn something or change"—to an asset informed approach that acknowledges that they know their child best. They may not discuss it or use the language I use, but they know some fundamental things about their child and their family that are assets. It is my job and my role to

hold up those assets, even if, I don't agree. It's our job to listen to what they say even if it's not a value that I hold."
(Shawn M. Bryant, Founding Director and Chief Learning Officer at Teaching Excellence Center)

Parents and families must be understood to be complex human beings and not defined by the trauma they experience. Trauma-responsive practice does not stigmatize, label or define people by their experiences of stress and trauma. Deficit thinking (words/terms used, stories told, beliefs held) is interrupted. Trauma and its impact are acknowledged honestly, however, it is never used to pathologize people. "Person-first"/"Identity-first" language and a strength-based approach is used by centering attention on the strengths, creativity, creative problem-solving, sources of coping, resilience and well-being and potential in parents, families and communities. Progress and accomplishments are celebrated.

A strength-based approach to family engagement begins with the assumption and belief that *all* children, parents and families have strengths, assets, sources of coping, resilience, creativity, brilliance and potential. We recognize families' expertise about their child and their profound contributions to their children's learning, development and well-being. Central to a strength-based approach is listening, observing and learning about the families in order to deepen our understanding of their beliefs, skills, knowledge, interests, relationships, cultural and linguistic practices, lived experiences and their hopes, dreams and goals for their children in our early learning programs.

Using a strength-based approach, we focus on families' strengths FIRST (versus their challenges, vulnerabilities, stressors and/or histories of trauma and oppression). A strength-based approach requires that we are open to adapting our policies and practices to be responsive to the specific families we are working with/serving at any point in time. We communicate "we see you;

we hear you, we care about you" and we will adapt our practices to be responsive to what we learn and know about you.

A strength-based approach does not mean we never talk about weaknesses. It does mean that we start from strengths to address weaknesses. It means uncovering and recognizing parents' and families' assets, resources, personal characteristics and relationships that can be mobilized to support them to address a need, to manage through an adverse circumstance and to heal when harmed. Strengths and assets can be used as a foundation from which to collaborate with families to address the problems and challenges they face. The vignette in the textbox below provides an example of a preschool teacher who helps parents honestly name their children's challenges but also encourages them that together they will look at the whole child in all their complex and wonderful humanity.

"I see your child and this negative thing that your kid is doing is not forever and it is not the sum of who your child is"—Muriel Johnson, lead preschool teacher, private preschool

Reading this vignette below, see if you can recognize how Muriel, when working with families, does not see their child through a deficit lens. Instead, she sees the "whole child" and says that a challenging behavior in the moment does not define a child or their family. She helps families to feel safe in her presence by communicating that she sees their children as complex people, not defined by their hardest moments of struggle and dysregulation. Muriel acts as a buffer to the stress that comes with parenting every day. Her interactions reduce parents' stress as you will see in the vignette below.

Every parent wants to know and feel like you like their child, bottom line. They want to feel like you see their child in a positive light. Even if, especially if, their child has difficulties. And so the way you talk to parents is huge. Anytime there are kids with behavioral issues and we have to meet with parents, I'm always included. I'm the buffer. The parents always say, "My kid feels uncomfortable here." I have a lot of compassion for them. One thing I always try to make sure parents understand is this: I see your child and this negative thing that your kid is doing is not forever and it is not the sum of who your child is. A lot of times parents will cry. They feel embarrassed, they feel ashamed. And I respond back in a reassuring way, "We're just having an experience with your child. This is part of parenthood. Our kids aren't perfect. I have my own stories." And sometimes I share personal stories with them. Being a parent is hard. It's not all joyful and fun. This is hard. You love them, but you will not always like your children.

I think one way I create good relationships with parents is throwing away the pretense that there is such thing as a perfect parent. I'm a teacher and I don't have perfect kids. It's all part of the journey of being human beings. And kids have a wide range of behaviors and personalities just like all humans do. And it's all okay and we are here in partnership to try to help them, support them, redirect them, whatever it is they need; we are a team and we are invested in this child. And this thing that your kid is doing, that you feel ashamed of and embarrassed about, it is not the sum of who he is. Do you see all this other great stuff that he does? We're going to work on the biting. It's not okay, but he's brilliant. He does all these other things. And so I feel like I really try to just be very frank with them and honor the challenge of parenting. I tell parents all the time, all the parents that you think have perfect kids and you envy, you don't know what goes on behind their doors. I'm not saying any names about anybody, but every parent has sat where you're sitting and divulges the same insecurities, the same shame you are feeling. You are thinking you're doing it so wrong and you see everyone doing it so right. It's an illusion. Do you think they are going to reveal and tell you their insecurities and what their kids did? Of course they're not.

When I reveal that these things are happening, my goal is to normalize it. I lay out, "I don't know if anyone's told you this or if you realize this, but this is actually normal and common." I tell parents to forgive themselves. "It's common to be mad at your kids. It's common to not like parenting. All those things. It doesn't mean you're a bad parent, that means you're human. Now what are we going to do? How are we going to problem solve this little issue that Monique's got? I've thought of some strategies. You tell me what strategies you're using at home. Let's try it out for a few weeks. And to tell you the truth, something might work for a week and then it won't work the next week. This is part of parenting." I'm always preparing them not to feel like it's a failure if there is regression but instead, that we are working through a process, we are on a journey. I have very comprehensive conversations with parents to make them feel pulled in and embraced. Hey, you can do this. It's not going to be easy and we don't have to lie and pretend about it. You don't have to tell me that she was biting because she was tired. Homegirl bites all the time. Homegirl's got an issue. She bites, not because she's tired. Let's throw that out the window. Forgive yourself. We're going to problem solve together.

Muriel illustrates the trauma-responsive principles Establishing Safety and Predictability and Acknowledging Strengths and Assets in the story above. She does this by humanizing the child and the process of parenting. Being a parent is hard. We all have uncertainty, challenges, moments of stress and times we don't know what to do. Like Muriel, we can buffer a parent's stress when we engage with them and create safety by helping them, by de-stigmatizing their struggles but never by blaming, criticizing or using language that shames them. Instead, trauma-responsive family engagement strives to build empathy with families and to buffer their stress through the power of trusting, attuned and responsive relationships and communication that reinforces our commitment to partner with them as early childhood professionals to work in collaboration to support their child's well-being. Muriel also reassures the parents that she sees many strengths in Monique. She reinforces that Monique is not the sum total of her biting behavior. Instead, her biting is a behavior they need to understand and work on together. Muriel, in partnering with the parents, is also acknowledging their strengths and assets and important role in supporting their child's development and learning.

Reflection/Discussion Questions

◆ When you have a child who is having challenges, what ways similar to Muriel do you approach a parent to help them feel safe to talk about it with you?

◆ How do you move yourself from your first reaction of "you need to fix your child's challenging behavior" to "we are going to solve this problem together?" And, I see your child's many strengths, not just this one behavior?

Before we can intentionally and consistently implement a strength-based approach in our work with families, we need to understand the barriers that prevent us from seeing and acknowledging their strengths and assets:

Deficit thinking is the most significant barrier that prevents early childhood professionals from using a strength-based approach in their work with parents and families.

What is deficit thinking? Deficit thinking includes beliefs, mindsets and assumptions about parents and family members, especially adults in historically minoritized groups including Black, Indigenous and People of Color, that see them through a "glass half empty" perspective, assuming they have individual and collective deficiencies that account for their hardships and the adversities they face. Deficit thinking is the root of all cycles of oppression. A minoritized group's "history, interests, needs and perspectives—their voices—are minimized or absent" (DiAngelo, 2016, p. 84). A deficit perspective is reflected in words/terms used, stories told and beliefs held about a minoritized group that are based on misinformation, partial information, misrepresentation and/or invisibility of their authentic lived experiences especially their strengths, capacities, accomplishments and histories of resistance and resilience.

> Whether a parent consciously recognizes it or not, every parent wants to know and feel like you like their child, bottom line. They want to feel like you see their child in a positive light. Even if their child has difficulties. And so the way you talk to parents is huge. Parents know when you don't like their children. They're not stupid. You can smile at them all day but they know—they feel— when you're not pleased with their child, when you are bothered by their child. That doesn't feel good as a parent, when it's coming from the person they leave their child with.
>
> (Muriel Johnson, lead preschool teacher,
> private preschool)

Research shows that in order to cultivate nurturing and trusting relationships with others, the ratio of focusing on strengths vs. deficits should be 5:1. That is, at least **five positive interactions for every negative one** (Lisitsa, 2012).

It takes effort and intentionality to disrupt deficit thinking and to focus on strengths.

One way to counter or disrupt deficit thinking is to invite parents and families to share their own stories about their children, their histories, their communities and their lived experiences— ideas, histories and narratives that are missing, invisible and/or inaccurate in the stories told and circulated about them.

"Have curiosity about the child and family"—Laura Rivas, Family Engagement Specialist, Berkeley Unified School District

> I have seen a shift from some teachers who have been willing to open up a space with a question and allow parents' voices to enter the room. Having a question be the first thing a teacher says is already centering the parents and families. This is especially important for White educators working with families of color. Let's say you are a White teacher and you have an immigrant family or maybe they're African American, or maybe you don't know much about them, but you're seeing some things in their child that's making you a bit worried. Instead of starting with your concerns, "I'm concerned about so-and-so" learn a little bit more about the child. **Have curiosity about the child and family.** "How was your weekend? How's it going with Miguel?" That is the approach I always try to take with families.

Laura shows how she collaborates with families with respect and a humility that prioritizes being curious, connecting and caring over showing her expert knowledge or coming directly to a family with concerns. She centers the relationship instead of allowing the focus to be on deficits and concerns. She acknowledges that trauma and stress do not define a family but that families are resourceful and resilient.

Acknowledging Parents and Families as the First and Most Important Teachers of their Children

When we work with families, we always say we partner with you and you are the experts in your family. You are the experts in your life, and we're here to help and support you and meet you where you're at.

(Aracely Nava, Family Engagement Coordinator, Child Development Resources)

The biggest lesson I learned working with so many families is that every time I'm talking to a family, I have to remind myself that I had a different experience growing up and I had a different childhood and I had a different experience and privileges than many of the families or my life may be a little bit more difficult than their lives. But the point is that I cannot judge them based on my experiences. So I have to without having judgment, because I will never know what they have been through or what they're going through. They are possibly reacting, the way that they are based on their experiences in their life. The only thing I can do is to listen to them and do my best to provide the resources that they may looking for. And to value their opinion. If they do not want my help, then they don't want it. I cannot force it on them. What I can do is to still be here for them whenever they're ready for us to support them.
(Rosalee Estrada, Family Engagement Specialist, Catholic Charities)

The belief that parents and families are their children's first and most important teachers is well represented in lists of best practices for high quality family engagement. This is a strength-based belief as it recognizes the critical role and contributions of families in young children's development, learning and well-being. This statement also communicates that families have valuable knowledge about their child and their family that early childhood professionals can and should learn about in order to be responsive in their work— whether they work directly with children and families or on their behalf in policy, research, advocacy, infrastructure or other roles.

Family engagement with a trauma-responsive lens means casting the spotlight of our attention on the strengths and the opportunity to partner to explore solutions between home and school. The easy path would be to direct and correct to achieve compliance. But this can be trauma-inducing if we insert our power over others. Instead, we want to approach the situation with humility and curiosity as reflected in the following vignette.

"That was my entry point to guide the staff to talk about how we could support Bisrat"—Shawn M. Bryant, Founding Director and Chief Learning Officer at Teaching Excellence Center

> Asset informed family engagement is finding out what are all the strengths and capacities that a family has, that a child has, that your early learning program has and using that knowledge to inform our practices. I will give you an example. There was a family at a preschool where I was coaching whose little boy, Bisrat would wake up from naptime in the afternoon viciously hungry. The teacher was frustrated and said to me, "He does this because he doesn't eat all day." And I asked, "What do you mean?" She replied, "He doesn't eat breakfast. He doesn't eat snack and he won't eat lunch. He says he doesn't want to eat any of these foods." Then, the other teacher spoke up, "You know, I sat down with him at the computer. I knew his family migrated here from Eretria so I Googled "Eritrea" to learn more about the foods they eat. When the pictures came up on the screen, Bisrat pointed at the pictures and said, "Oh, we eat that! We eat that! We eat that! We eat that!" And in my mind I was thinking, "Okay, is there a way to talk to someone and find out if we can have some of these foods available for him?"
>
> All of this is family engagement because Bisrat is coming from his family and understanding his family helps us understand his behavior. And the classroom team has knowledge and expertise that could support this family. Acknowledging these two points was my entry point to guide the staff to talk about how we could support Bisrat. Something as simple as a meal goes back to the context and conditions from his home. The solution wasn't asking

his parents to send food every day. That's the easy way out to say, "He's not eating anything so you will need to send food from home so that he can eat." Instead, it's how we form a real relationship with the family to say, "Here's what's going on. We would like to explore some opportunities to get him to eat here. We're going to try to hold his lunch and when he wakes up, to offer it to him and maybe have someone sit with him. If that doesn't work, we're going to try something else. He showed us pictures on the screen of foods he says he eats at home. If some food came from home, would he eat that?" We would explore with the family what the possible solutions are. To me, that's family engagement. We have this traditional notion, or I like to call it the 19th-century notion, that doing these things would spoil children. It's not spoiling, it's actually getting this child's needs met so he has an optimal experience in preschool. Making these types of connections isn't just child centered, it's family centered.

Shawn did not jump quickly to an easy fix to this problem. Working with families and children requires that we pause, reflect and slow down to explore the situation. The first trauma-responsive principle we see in this vignette is Focusing on Strengths and Assets. Shawn was able to look beyond the initial presentation of the child having challenging behaviors (not eating all day) to the meaning behind the challenges. He asked himself, "what is this child not eating communicating to us?" He was able uncover the child had familiar foods at home and the new foods being presented did not feel safe, predictable or comfortable for the child. Shawn went on to explore the next trauma-responsive principle, Create Power Sharing Partnerships where collaboration and reciprocity are emphasized—listening and learning that is bidirectional and based in respect, humility, curiosity and openness to challenge dominant "taken for granted" assumptions about universal "best" practices and policy solutions. Shawn suggested that the teacher share power with the family by exploring solutions instead of just telling them what to do so that a bridge could be created between the cultural norms at school and that of home. Using these principles to guide practice does not spoil the child but instead, supports the child to thrive in the context of a culturally responsive approach to meeting his needs.

Reflection/Discussion Questions

+ In your work with parents and families, can you think of a time when you had to create a bridge between cultural norms at school at those at home?
+ How did you use a culturally responsive approach to meet the needs of the child and create a bridge between both home and school?
+ Were you able to take steps to create bidirectional communication with the family that promoted a power sharing partnership to explore solutions?

Being trauma informed and responsive means being aware of your power. When you are in a position of power it can automatically trigger others without you even doing or saying anything. Recognizing this power is important. As traumatic experiences involve a loss of power and control resulting in feelings of helplessness, terror and often, hopelessness, trauma-responsive and resilience building practices focus on building relational connections and scanning for strengths and prioritizing connection over delivering content or directing others.

Note

1 See Nadal's (2014) *Guide to Responding to Microaggressions* and Haslam's (2019) *Guide to Interrupting Bias: Calling Out vs. Calling in for Helpful Suggestions.*

References

DiAngelo, R. (2016). *What does it mean to be White? Developing White racial literacy* (Revised ed.). New York: Peter Lang.

Haslam, R. E. (2019). Interrupting bias: Calling out vs. calling in. Seed the Way LLC. Retrieved from www.seedtheway.com/uploads/8/8/0/0/8800499/calling_in_calling_out__3_.pdf.

Lisitsa, E. (2012). The positive perspective: Dr. Gottman's magic ratio! [Web log post]. Retrieved from www.gottmanblog.com/2012/12/the-positive-perspective-dr-gottmans.html.

Nadal, K. (2014). A guide to responding to microaggressions. *CUNY Forum*, *2*(1), 71–76. Retrieved from https://advancingjustice-la.org/sites/default/files/ELAMICRO%20A_Guide_to_Responding_to_Microaggressions.pdf.

Singh, A. (2019). *The racial healing handbook: Practical activities to help you challenge privilege, confront systemic racism, and engage in collective healing*. Oakland, CA: New Harbinger.

Wing Sue, D., Capodilupo, C., Torino, G., Bucceri, J., Holder, A., Nadal, K., & Esquilin. M. (2007). Racial microaggressions in everyday life: Implications for counseling. *The American Psychologist*, *62*(4), 271–286.

7

CORE PRINCIPLE: Provide Opportunities for Agency and Control

My organizing background has been so helpful to gather with families and to provide them with the space where they can raise questions and concerns and then channel their energy to action. I value having families themselves come up with solutions. What they would like to see. I want families to brainstorm and hear ideas from each other and from themselves. And then we work together to plan what the advocacy is going to be at the level of the school and then at the level of the district.

(Laura Rivas, Family Engagement Specialist,
Berkeley Unified School District)

As traumatic experiences involve a loss of power and control resulting in feelings of helplessness, terror and often, hopelessness, trauma-responsive practices support parents and families to have opportunities for agency and control. This is often described as "voice and choice." Trauma-responsive environments support parents and families to

DOI: 10.4324/9781003127666-8

have opportunities to provide input to inform the decisions that impact them (e.g., policies, processes and procedures), to make choices and participate in creating mutually agreed upon goals, and to feel a sense of control in communication, interactions and within early learning environments.

There are a wide range of ways this principle looks in practice. The vignette below highlights one example of family engagement where an elementary school Family Engagement Specialist worked in collaboration with Latinx parents at her school—concerned about proposed funding cuts that would severely impact the quality of their children's education—to use their voices and within the structure of the system to advocate and push back against the proposed cuts. The Family Engagement Specialist sees these parents as having strengths and capacities to be effective advocates and she guides them, and shares power with them, so they have agency and control in learning how to express their opinions to school and district leaders and School Board members; an experience that she described as transformative for them.

"That experience really changed them"—Laura Rivas, Family Engagement Specialist, Berkeley Unified School District

> It started in the English learners advocacy committee and that group meets every month. We had several meetings and parents were rallying behind funding cuts that were going to be happening at our school. The parents were concerned about the impact that the funding cuts would have on their children. They asked, "What can we do?" And I responded, "Let's think together." And some parents suggested that they write a letter. I asked them if anyone had invited the principal. Their response was, "No, she doesn't listen to us. How can we get her to listen?" I suggested that we invite her to the next meeting, emphasizing, "we want her to be with us together. She has power. We can offer her the questions that you would

like to ask about the cuts and she can ask her superiors. If they don't get back to her, then we can take it to the next step and go to the School Board." Some parents were ready to go to the School Board right off the bat but after pausing to reflect on the best course of action, they decided to try to partner with our principal. They came up with questions they wanted to ask of the principal. We were able to rally all of the parents behind this effort to get our principal to partner with us.

Before the principal came to the meeting, I had already talked with her and she was prepared. She expressed her concerns with me, "They're just going to chew me up." I told her, "No, they don't want to fight with you. They'll have your back. You just have to be there and you have to listen to them." And so she took a risk and showed up, heard everybody and she reassured them that if she did not hear back from her district leaders by the following week, she would let them (the parents) know. The principal did receive a response from the district leaders but it was kind of a lukewarm response. So we (the parents and I) decided to go forward to the School Board meeting. For many parents, it was their first time speaking at a School Board meeting. For some it was their first time ever speaking publicly. They decided to work on their speeches together. We wrote them out in advance of the meeting (except one dad, who decided to do his on the fly). They told me what they wanted to say, I wrote it down for them and then we edited it together. We had four parents lined up to speak, but we had about 25 parents show up. It was really beautiful. All the parents who spoke that night were immigrant, Latinx parents; some of them spoke in Spanish and they had an interpreter. **That experience really changed them.** I have seen how afterwards they were not as afraid.

As Laura's work with these Latinx families reflects, true family engagement acknowledges parents as experts with valuable insight on how to transform early childhood programs, schools and school systems. Parents are recognized as leaders who, working in partnership with early childhood professionals, can intervene and advocate on behalf of their children not only to inspire change within their child's agency or program, but also to work in solidarity with larger movements for justice and equity in our society. Laura partners with parents and centers their voices and agency, a trauma-responsive practice that disrupts our inequitable history of silencing the contributions of families of color.

The next vignette describes how Jonathan Iris-Wilbanks, a Child Life Specialist, is working to create trauma-responsive environments in a hospital setting. As you read through the story, identify how Jonathan's beliefs and actions reflect the essence of this principle, Provide Opportunities for Agency and Control, in context:

"I call the families and give them a little of that emotional prep"—Jonathan Iris-Wilbanks, Child Life Specialist

> I get a list at the beginning of the week of the upcoming medical procedures and the highly stressful procedures for young children. I **call the families** and have a quick five minute conversation about what to bring and what they might see and walk them through what to expect when they arrive; essentially I **give them a little emotional prep**. For some children, if they have sensory processing challenges, we explore whether it is safe for them to wear their own pajamas. I talk with the doctors, "Is this child's type of pajamas going to be safe in an MRI machine?" Because some stretchy elastic material actually has metal in it and it could heat up and hurt the child. I try to find ways for the children to have a chance to wear at least one piece of their own clothing. Something as seemingly small as having the opportunity to wear their own socks can help a child feel an increased sense of safety and control while going through a stressful procedure in the hospital.

Jonathan used two trauma-responsive principles in the example above. The first is Establishing Safety and Predictability. By calling the parents and explaining the expectations and the steps in the process, he helps to create a sense of predictability and reduces uncertainty for the parents. When the parents know what to expect, it can reduce their anxiety allowing them to feel a sense of safety and reduce their stress levels. In turn, it may increase their ability to be present and co-regulate their own child's anxiety. Jonathan's practice also reflects the trauma-responsive principle, Provide Opportunities for Agency and Control, as he offers choices for both the child and family. Small moments where we have choices and a voice to express our opinions can increase peoples' feelings of control which in turn, can reduce feelings of powerlessness and stress.

Reflection/Discussion Questions

- ◆ Can you remember an example of when you invited a family or parent to make small choices or to have a voice?
- ◆ Have you taken any steps to help families and/or children feel safe in times of uncertainty or stress?

Asking for Consent: Parents and Families as "Invited Guests"

Bill Ketterer, author of, *Reducing Anger and Violence in Schools* (2019), explains that an important way early childhood providers can build trust with parents and families in the early learning setting is to consider **the concept of becoming an invited guest.** The idea of the "invited guest" is based on a belief that building trust with parents and families—especially if they have histories of trauma including difficult experiences interacting with educational systems—will be enhanced when educators *ask permission to be part of the parent's/family member's life.* That is, to help the family feel as if they have choices about how things will proceed in the relationships and to allow them **the chance to withdraw emotionally** if necessary. In essence, to be an "invited guest" is to acknowledge that processing or otherwise discussing sensitive topics—e.g., feelings, behavior—requires consent and should only be done after the early childhood provider asks permission. This small but simple act of requesting consent to open a conversation with a family about a topic that may be difficult for a parent and evoke strong emotions, provides them with agency by *allowing them to have a way out.* Although it may seem counterintuitive, the invited guest concept is one of the best ways to build confidence and safety as trust is enhanced "when people have the ability to leave" (Ketterer, 2019). How does granting permission to "leave" build trust? By...

- ♦ Communicating messages to the parents and families that they have choices
- ♦ Reducing the power differential between educators and families
- ♦ Allowing opportunities for withdrawing
- ♦ Using family input to inform decisions and processes

What does "asking for consent" look like? Requesting to be an invited guest in the life of a parent/family might sound like:

- ♦ Your child said something in class today that I'd like to share with you. Is this a good time to discuss this with you?
- ♦ Would you be willing to meet with us/me about your child's preferences for different foods?
- ♦ I want to share some things about your child in our classroom. May I share some of my observations with you?
- ♦ How much time do you have for our meeting?
- ♦ Where is best location for you to meet?
- ♦ Where would you like me to sit?
- ♦ Should I take my shoes off (when entering a home)?

Dr. Ketterer suggests that early childhood providers think of the invited guest concept like an **invitation for tea**. He explains:

The parents may at first want a cup of tea, so to speak, but then later they decide that they don't. Of course, at a tea party, if a person doesn't like their tea, they can stop drinking it at any time. The same goes with discussions at school about behavior, concerns, family issues etc. *We want to be respectful of the parent and family member's right to change their mind about having that "cup of tea."*

(p. 87)

Communicating to parents and family members that you understand, acknowledge and will respect their voice and agency in the relationship is simply making transparent the power that families always have to disengage from educational settings and processes. Many parents find ways to withdraw emotionally and physically—and not to engage or to stop participating in an educational program in an authentic or collaborative way—when they feel inherently unsafe, unwelcome and perceive that they do not have control in determining how and when they participate.

Reflection/Discussion Questions

◆ What is your reaction to the idea of being an invited guest and taking a stance of "asking permission" in your work with parents and families?

◆ How can this concept of being an invited guest influence the way you interact with a parent or family? How can it help you build trust with families?

◆ Thinking about a meeting with a parent/family, how would you do the following:
  • Invite them to a meeting
  • Set up the meeting space
  • Welcome them to the meeting
  • Set the agenda (in advance or during)
  • Start of the meeting and determine the time, agenda and next steps
  • Balance the discussion between your agenda items and theirs
  • Help them feel safe to offer disagreements or different ideas
  • Offer opportunities for their input

Following is an example of using the concept of the "Invited Guest" in an early childhood program.

Javier Diaz is a home visitor for a Head Start Program in Texas. He visits families weekly and provides parenting education and support services. He shares with us how he uses this concept of the "invited guest":

> Two days before my appointment with a family, I send a friendly text asking if they are still free for our appointment and if the time still works for them. I also invite them to feel free to share any topics, concerns or questions they may have. I make sure they have a choice to send this information in advance in writing or, if they prefer, to wait for the meeting so they are able to choose which way to communicate based on what they are most comfortable with. I have found some families do better by sending their thoughts in writing in advance but are not as comfortable when I am with them in person. The day of the meeting, I send off one more text as a friendly reminder telling them that I am on my way. When I arrive at the family's home for a visit, I knock in case a child is sleeping. When they open the door, I ask if they prefer that I take off my shoes. In the beginning, I always ask where they prefer for me to sit. We start off every meeting with me asking them, "Tell me what is on your mind this week. How are you doing?" This open ended question allows them to lead the conversation with topics that are important to them.

Javier uses this strategy of the "invited guest" to illustrate the trauma-responsive principle of Providing Opportunities for Agency and Control. This principle is often described as giving people "voice and choice" which can provide a sense of control in an environment. The more stress and chaos we feel in our lives, the more we can feel out of control and this can be expounded when it triggers past feelings of trauma. When Javier asks the family for consent or offers them with choices, he provides them with opportunities to have a sense of power and control in the interaction which can significantly help adults to calm their stress response systems and maintain or return to a state of regulation.

Reflection/Discussion Questions

♦ Have you ever had someone come into your familiar environment/home and they acted as if they were an "invited guest"? How did that feel for you?

♦ Have you ever entered the home or the environment of someone else and you acted as if you were the "invited guest" using the concept above? What did you notice?

CORE PRINCIPLE: Use Culturally, Linguistically and Individually Responsive Practices

Trauma-responsive practice acknowledges that there are many different culturally informed practices and approaches for responding to, and coping with, stress and trauma as well as for fostering health, healing and wellness for parents, families, groups and communities. Responses to stress, trauma and healing should be generated and/ or informed by the children and families impacted by the practices so they are aligned with their cultural and spiritual beliefs, values and practices and the primary languages that are familiar to them.

Culture is a broad concept that refers to deep-rooted customs, values, beliefs, languages, social norms and practices shared among a group of people that may be transmitted across generations (Rogoff, 2003, 2011). According to the cultural psychologist Barbara Rogoff, our lives can be considered coherent constellations of cultural practices that may dynamically change over time, over social and environmental settings and across generations (Rogoff & Angelillo, 2002; Rogoff, 2003,

2011). Even without our conscious awareness, **culture plays a significant and complex role in shaping how we think, believe, behave and engage with the world including how we learn, perceive and respond to stress and trauma and how we heal** (National Academies of Sciences, Engineering, and Medicine, 2018). Guarino, Soares, Konnath, Clervil and Bassuk (2009) emphasize the connections between culture, trauma and healing:

> Traumatic events happen to people from all racial and ethnic backgrounds, and the brain's response to trauma is consistent for all trauma survivors. However, culture plays a significant role in the types of trauma that may be experienced, the risk for continued trauma, how survivors manage and express their experiences, and which supports and interventions are most effective. Violence and trauma have different meanings across cultures, and healing takes place within one's own cultural "meaning-making" system.
>
> (p. 27)

How Do Culture and Language Influence Peoples' Experiences of Stress, Trauma, Mental Health and Healing?

Culture wires our brains. Although more research is needed to examine the relationships between culture, stress and trauma, several studies have documented how different cultural beliefs and experiences influence:

- ◆ Perceptions of threat and danger
- ◆ How trauma-related memories are stored and retrieved in our brains and bodies
- ◆ Peoples' physiological arousal—that is, the processes involved in the activation of the stress response system (fight, flight, freeze)
- ◆ Peoples' recovery times after a stressful interaction or situation

- ◆ The emotional states induced from a stressful or traumatic experience
- ◆ And peoples' perceptions and responses to others' distress (Cheon et al., 2013; Liddell & Jobson, 2016; Park & Huang, 2010).

These research studies, from the field of Cultural Neuroscience, highlight why it is so important that we build awareness of the cultural values, perceptions and beliefs that influence how we perceive and interact with parents and families; and to the extent possible, to learn about the cultural perspectives of the children and families we work with as well as those of our colleagues. Imagine a home visitor saying, "This family never hugs their children, it makes me wonder why there is so little love in this family," because she was raised to see love through hugs and words of affirmation. If we are not careful to question our assumptions and to realize that culture impacts everything we observe, believe and do and that there is not "one" right way (Rogoff, 2003; e.g., there are multiple ways to show love and cultures vary in this expression), we can too easily judge, stigmatize, alienate and harm the families we are intending to support.

The only way to create early childhood programs that implement culturally, linguistically and individually responsive practices is to build a solid foundation of trust with the parents and families you serve. Why? Because our families come from so many different cultural backgrounds, they often speak a range of languages and the community contexts where they live, work and play are so unique and diverse. And so, as shared in many ways throughout this book, we have to begin by listening and learning from them. However, they are only going to share with us when they feel respected, welcome and safe. It is important to translate materials into the home languages of our families. Additionally, it is important to communicate in ways that feel safe or that are accessible. Some families have so much stress that filling out a form and turning it in is not possible, not because of the language translation, but because of the focal attention that is not available due to the high levels of overwhelm. Building trust with families starts by helping them to feel safe in our presence and within our programs. Only when they no longer detect threat, will their cortex be open enough so they can "hear" the messages we are sending.

The following vignette describes how one early childhood professional, who had built trust with parents and families over many years in one urban community, was able to use her relationship to help families move from fear and skepticism to interest and openness in their response to a government program. Claudia's story below highlights the importance of building trust through a culturally responsive lens.

> Culturally and linguistically responsive family engagement refers to practices that honor the role of families' culture, language, and experience in supporting their children's learning and development. When families are invited to share information about their children and their experiences, providers gain a better understanding of children's cultural and linguistic backgrounds and learning preferences...Cultural and linguistic responsiveness also requires that systems, programs, and personnel recognize their own cultures and biases, and work to value differing cultures and languages.
>
> (USDHHS, 2016, p. 4)

Her program uses a traditional parent involvement/parent education approach. However, they identify several family-community liaisons who are trusted in their local communities and who support communication between schools and families with different cultural and linguistic backgrounds.

"We created pods of families"—Claudia Medina, Supervisor, Family and Community Engagement Programs, Alameda Unified School District

> Something that I invested early on was having parent education programs like School Smarts that has been an essential program for me to build capacity and rapport with families. We provide these programs in

different languages in our district to help build families' understanding of their relationship with schools. What will their children learn? How do they know who's who in schools, how do they navigate the public school system? And how are decisions made? We translated what was already in English into Chinese and Spanish, Tagalog and Vietnamese and Arabic. From there **we created pods of families** with family-community liaisons who are the bridge between the school and our families. I have a Chinese family-community liaison, as well as an Arabic speaking, Vietnamese speaking, Chinese speaking, Mongolian speaking and Spanish speaking liaison. Whenever we have parent events, I go to the liaisons and then they share out the information through Facebook, WeChat, WhatsApp and other formats because they know how families are going to connect. This has been a very big outreach success for me, leveraging these relationships so I can reach families who speak multiple languages.

Reflection/Discussion Questions
   ◆   How do you dismantle top down systems and instead, create power-sharing partnerships that help support families to feel safe to share their voices and to provide input on policies, programs or changes that will impact them and/or their children?
   ◆   When you are working with families, how do you build "trusted partners" or "liaisons" within your community who are responsive to the cultures, the language and the community's needs?

Rosalie Estrada, a Family Resource Center supervisor, and her staff also strive to work with families in a manner that is responsive to their diverse cultural ways of knowing and aligned with their home languages. She explains that central to their work is learning to notice and stop themselves from making assumptions about parents and families.

"The last thing we want to do is to make assumptions"—Rosalie Estrada, Family Resource Center Supervisor, Catholic Charities

We are so lucky that we are a very diverse center. We have families from Vietnam, from Mexico, from the rest of Latin American. We have families from India, from all over the world. And as you know, every single country has different cultures and different traditions, and people see things from different points of view. So **the last thing we want to do is to make assumptions**. We don't want parents to be scared of us or to think that we are here to impose things on them. As one example, we have one family from Mexico that I believed needed support with food. But I was aware that for some families, if a parent asks for food, their belief is that they've failed as a provider for their family. So, I had a conversation with the father in this family and he was asking me a bunch of questions. I knew this family needed food because I also have a connection with the afterschool program and mom had shared this with the director. I also knew that the father would never accept food as a handout because it would be like accepting that he was not providing for his family. So, I took a different approach and asked him if there was anything he was interested in at the Family Resource Center. He replied, "I would like to volunteer here." And I said, "Perfect. We have the food bank distribution and we always need help." So I asked him if he could volunteer to help us at the food bank. In exchange for volunteering, he would take food home at the end of his shift. He was pleased to be earning the food in exchange for work. And I was grateful that we could find a way to work with him in a manner that respected his cultural beliefs and also provided meaningful support to his family.

This is not easy! Family engagement is not an exact science with a clear pathway outlining the best way to engage. We must give ourselves grace and room to grow but also be willing to take risks and to learn new ways of seeing and approaching our work. You may not always agree with parents' cultural viewpoints at times and this can make things complicated. But to listen and make an attempt to understand and empathize with a family's cultural beliefs is an important part of building trust, creating a sense of safety and welcome and supporting the child to experience continuity between home and the early childhood program. There are times that programs may need to diverge from a family's cultural viewpoint or cultural routines (e.g., harsh forms of punishment, separating genders, etc.) and when this is the case, we attempt to listen first, then to communicate to families the "why" behind our program's policy or practice in a way that does not evaluate or judge their cultural beliefs and practices.

Culturally and linguistically responsive family engagement practices communicate to young children, parents and family members that their family identities are seen and valued *and* that families in early childhood programs have a diverse range of backgrounds, structures, cultural beliefs and practices and speak a wide range of languages.

How many of the following STRATEGIES are you using in your program? (Adapted from: Teaching Tolerance, 2018):

Use Inclusive and Accessible Language. Use language that is inclusive of all families in your writing and communication. Instead of beginning emails/announcements or notes home with the phrase, "Dear Parents" use "Dear Families" instead. Review language for assumptions about a family's resources, family traditions and cultural practices, political affiliations or other life circumstances. Additionally, increase the ability for busy and stressed families and families whose primary language is not English to understand the key messages in your written communication. The following websites offer guidance on how to keep your writing simple, clear and easy to understand for parents and families:

◆ www.plainlanguage.gov/guidelines/
◆ www.cms.gov/Outreach-and-Education/Outreach/
  WrittenMaterialsToolkit/index.html
◆ https://childcareta.acf.hhs.gov/sites/default/files/
  public/ce-websiteguide-508_3-16-18.pdf.

Source: USDHHS (2018, p. 16)

Recognize Families' Key Relationships. We all need to make a point of learning about the important relationships in each child's life—including those who may not be legal parents or guardians—and involving them as appropriate. This may include welcoming biological, adoptive, and step-parents as well as primary caregivers, such as grandparents, other adult family members, kinship caregivers and foster or resource parents and biological or nonbiological, chosen or circumstantial family members (ECLKC, n.d.) to be part of our early learning programs and services.

Use Home Language Whenever Possible. Because language is central to families' lives, identities and daily functioning, early childhood programs should communicate with parents in their home languages as much as possible. Translating materials and providing interpreting services in families' home languages supports them to engage with the program as partners. See vignette below for an example of one early learning program successfully doing this for linguistically diverse families in their community.

Gather Important Information at Enrollment or Throughout the Year. Early childhood educators can gather valuable information about children by connecting with parents and guardians at enrollment and also throughout the year. Asking family members about their children's strengths, challenges and lives outside of school—as well as about their own hopes and fears for their children's caregiving and education—provides important background, sets a collaborative tone and allows classroom practice to reflect children's and families' identities.

Integrate Family and Community Wisdom. Our families possess tremendous experiential wisdom on issues related to identity, culture, history, oppression and justice. Parents, caregivers, families, neighbors, community leaders and knowledge keepers/elders have important stories to share about their lived experiences, cultural rituals and practices and their perspectives. Family and community wisdom brings to life diverse cultural ways of knowing, diverse histories and experiences of historical and cultural trauma as well as cultural assets, and individual as well as collective forms of resilience, resistance, coping and healing. Hearing from our family members who have lived through decades of change and/or participated in social justice movements can inspire children's development, learning, sense of belonging and well-being. Children and families bring essential cultural and linguistic knowledge with them. Making room to share this knowledge and make it visible and valued in our early learning programs is an important foundation of trauma-responsive practice and supports children's healthy identity development by deepening their positive sense of self and connection to family and community. Additionally, when children hear stories about other children's families and experiences, they are supported at a young age to expand their awareness and develop respect for diverse groups, cultures and communities.

Lotus Bloom Family Resource Centers
(www.lotusbloomfamily.org/story.html)

Lotus Bloom is a network of three **multicultural family resource centers** built in Oakland, California from the ground up. Lotus Bloom FRCs strive to become "places in the community where families can celebrate their cultural, linguistic, and unique diversity, and appreciate and respect their collective differences and commonalities. ... spaces that are vibrant thriving hubs for families to gather, learn, and grow." Lotus Bloom is committed to culturally and linguistically responsive work with families. They provide multicultural playgroups, parent workshops and cafes and community events. See the following videos created for families to see examples of their cultural, linguistic and contextually responsive communication with young children and their families:

♦ Drumming for Justice with Mr. Pablo www.youtube.com/watch?v=RxhuzactFNQ&feature=youtu.be
♦ Hip Hop Circle Time with Mr. Rha www.youtube.com/watch?v=xro38-rIfng&feature=youtu.be
♦ Let's Go on an Urban Walk with Mr. Rha www.youtube.com/watch?v=I687rWxgtRA&feature=youtu.be

Tandem, Partners in Early Learning is a nonprofit organization working at the intersection of social justice and early childhood education. An important goal for Tandem is to provide culturally and linguistically responsive materials that families can use to engage children in joyful conversations. Tandem's book collection, comprising 1,300 titles in 21 languages, is at the center of the organization's work and curating special book collections for Oakland's diverse families is a key program element. Tandem works in collaboration with several school- and center-based early learning programs and community partners (like Refugee and Immigrant Transitions, for example) to connect with and serve young children and families.

Paola Bea is an Early Learning Specialist who works for Tandem and acts as a liaison between her agency and their community partners. As an example of her work, Paola recently collaborated with an early childhood teacher, Antonia, who told her that she had some new Mayan families, recently arrived from Guatemala, who speak Mam, an Indigenous language. Paola asked Antonia if she could find storybooks in Mam that she could share with these families. Paola explains how Tandem works with families to help in the selection and vetting of storybooks for their various collections.

Vignette: "Our goal is that all families have a good book sharing experience with their children"—Paola Bea, Early Learning Specialist, Tandem Partners for Early Learning

> I knew of two families who were Mam speakers and readers. I asked them if they would be willing to review children's books translated into Mam if I was able to locate any. I explained that we would ask them to read the storybooks and then share their feedback. The types of questions we ask families to think about when reviewing books in their home languages: "Is it translated in the way you speak or read in your home language?" "In your perspective, is this story appropriate for young children?" and "Does the book reflect your culture in the way that you want to be talking about your culture with your children?" If they approve a book, then we add it to our collection. **Our goal is that all families have a good book sharing experience with their children.** And we believe that if we send home books in a language that nobody speaks in the home, that is less likely to happen. We learn about the needs of our parents and families from our community partners. A lot of our sites have Arabic speaking families and Dari speaking families. We also have families from Cambodia, Laos and recently many are arriving from Eritrea. Yesterday, I was at a preschool and a teacher said, "I have a child from Vietnam. Do you have any Vietnamese storybooks?"
>
> We believe it is really important for us to get families' perspectives about whether the books we find are the kinds of books that they want to be reading with their children. For example, there is a book called, Festival of Colors, which is about the Indian festival of Holi. This is

the kind of book that I feel is written from a White perspective. The author is Indian, but it is written for a non-Indian audience. So it's really important that we engage with families in reading and reviewing books as we create our collections. Their work is so important and we want this partnership with the linguistically diverse families in our community to become central to all of our programs. We are currently working on what kind of compensation or recognition we would like to provide the families for the time they give to review books. One idea we had, after the adults complete the tasks of evaluating the books is to create an opportunity for the community of families (e.g., the Mam speaking families) to come together to receive the books and at that event, we would give recognition and acknowledgment to the reviewers. I know the families really appreciate receiving books in their home language. When they look at a book their child brings home and they see that it was written in their home language, it really makes them smile.

Tandem offers a beautiful illustration of their use of the trauma-responsive principle, Implementing Culturally, Linguistically and Contextually Responsive Practices in early childhood. They honor the strengths and cultural and linguistic assets of the families they serve and they create partnerships with the families in ways that give them real decision-making power to influence the program's goals and processes and ensure they reflect their values, beliefs, practices and languages. When a child can see their family, culture and language reflected in their early learning environment, it validates and values who they are in the world. It creates an environment of inclusion and belonging and this is trauma responsive.

Reflection/Discussion Questions

- ◆ Thinking of this principle, in what ways have you reached out to families to get their perspective, input or feedback on the books and/or materials being considered for your program?

◆ Tandem uses three criteria for vetting new materials for a classroom. Is this something you might consider for your program?
  • Is it translated in the way you speak or read in your home language?
  • In your perspective, is this story appropriate for young children?
  • Does the book reflect your culture in the way that you want to be talking about your culture with your children?

References

Cheon, B. K., Im, D. M., Harada, T., Kim, J. S., Mathur, V. A., Scimeca, J. M., …Chiao, J. Y. (2013). Cultural modulation of the neural correlates of emotional pain perception: The role of other-focusedness. *Neuropsychologia*, 51(7), 1177–1186.

Early Childhood Learning and Knowledge Center (ECLKC). (n.d.). *Parent involvement and family engagement. For early childhood professionals*. Office of Head Start, Administration of Children and Families. Retrieved from https://eclkc.ohs.acf.hhs.gov/sites/default/files/pdf/parent-involvement-family-engagement-forprofessionals.pdf.

Guarino, K., Soares, P., Konnath, K., Clervil, R. & Bassuk, E. (2009). *Trauma-informed organizational toolkit*. Rockville, MD: Center for Mental Health Services, Substance Abuse and Mental Health Services Administration, and the Daniels Fund, the National Child Traumatic Stress Network, and the W.K. Kellogg Foundation. Retrieved from www.homeless.samhsa.gov and www.familyhomelessness.org.

Ketterer, B. (2019). *Reducing anger and violence in schools: An evidence based approach*. New York, NY: Routledge.

Liddell, B. J., & Jobson, L. (2016). The impact of cultural differences in self-representation on the neural substrates of posttraumatic stress disorder. *European Journal of Psychotraumatology*, 7(30464). https://doi.org/10.3402/ejpt.v7.30464.

National Academies of Sciences, Engineering, and Medicine, The (2018). How people learn II: Learners, contexts, and cultures. Retrieved from www.nap.edu/catalog/24783/how-people-learn-ii-learners-contexts-and-cultures.

Park, D., & Huang, C. (2010). Culture wires the brain: A cognitive neuroscience perspective. Perspectives on Psychological Science, 5(4), 391–400. https://doi.org/10.1177/1745691610374591.

Rogoff, B. (2003). The cultural nature of human development. Oxford: Oxford University Press.

Rogoff, B. (2011). Developing destinies: A Mayan midwife and town. Oxford: Oxford University Press.

Rogoff, B., & Angelillo, C. (2002). Investigating the coordinated functioning of multifaceted cultural practices in human development. Human Development, 45(4), 211–225.

Teaching Tolerance (2018). Critical practices for anti-bias education. Retrieved from www.tolerance.org/magazine/publications/critical-practices-for-antibias-education.

U.S. Department of Health and Human Services & U.S. Department of Education. (2016). Policy statement on family engagement: From the early years to the early grades. Retrieved from www2.ed.gov/about/inits/ed/earlylearning/files/policy-statement-on-family-engagement.pdf.

U.S. Department of Health and Human Services, Administration for Children and Families, Office of Head Start, National Center on Parent, Family, and Community Engagement. (USDHHS) (2018). Key indicators of high-quality family engagement for quality rating improvement systems. https://childcareta.acf.hhs.gov/sites/default/files/public/indicators-final-508.pdf.

8

CORE PRINCIPLE: Promote Coping, Resilience, Healing and Wellness

To me, resilience is when individuals are able to overcome their challenges and stressors and adapt to changes that are unforeseen. It is the ability to cope despite challenges and to learn from experiences. Being trauma-responsive and healing-centered is looking at the whole individual, not just focusing on their trauma, but understanding an individual within their family, their culture and their background and supporting them in a comprehensive and holistic way, in all aspects of who they are, not just targeting and focusing on their trauma.

(Aracely Nava, Family Engagement Coordinator, Child Development Resources)

Central to trauma-responsive family engagement practice is actively building the skills, knowledge and dispositions necessary for coping, resilience, healing and wellness. Examples include strengthening such social and emotional

DOI: 10.4324/9781003127666-9

capacities as self-awareness, body awareness, sensory and emotional literacy, self-regulation (emotional and behavioral), relationship skills, problem-solving and decision making. These skills improve parents' and families' abilities to cope, build resilience and heal and for educators to strengthen resilience in their work with parents and families impacted by trauma.

Resilience is seen with children and adults who are succeeding, even excelling, despite incredibly difficult circumstances.

We want to create environments that are not only trauma-responsive but also intentionally build resilience and support healing for parents and families. Creating environments that are safe, predictable and focus on building relational connections may be one of the greatest proactive interventions we can do to build their resilience. We cannot create resilient environments without healthy early childhood providers who intentionally promote their own self-care, self-awareness and self-regulation. It is all interconnected and when we make one small change toward health and wellness, the ripple effect is significant. Although there are many ways that coping and resilience can be intentionally planned for and strengthened, it is critical to name that the lack of resources in early childhood is an ever-present barrier and challenge.

What Factors Support Children and Adults to Cope, Heal and Build Resilience?

♦ **Having consistent, supportive and responsive relationships.** Caring attuned responsive relationships are the most important factor to buffer stress, prevent short- and long-term harm resulting from trauma *and* to support children's and adults' healing. Perry (2017) reinforces the power of relationships to buffer stress and heal, *"Just as a traumatic experience can alter a life in* *an instant, so too can a therapeutic encounter.* The more we can provide each other these moments of simple, human connection—even a brief nod or a moment of eye contact—the more we'll be able to heal those who have suffered traumatic experiences" (pp. 308–309).

In addition to building relationships between early childhood professionals and parents and families, essential to family engagement is supporting *family-to-family activities and other social networking opportunities* to foster a sense of community for families within early learning programs and to the larger community to strengthen their access to supports and resources (USDHHS, 2018). The story below highlights how one program is using a two-generation approach to build relationships between the children and families they serve and elders in the community. Notice how this program builds relationships in ways that buffers stress, promotes resilience for the seniors, parents and families and preserves the cultural traditions, languages and historical ways of knowing that are a source of strength—a community cultural asset—for everyone.

> We have one amazing group called **Las Quinceaneras or Generation to Generation**. They are a group of adults 55 years and older. They meet at the Family Resource Center on Tuesdays and Fridays every single week. And the idea was for them to reconnect back to society and not to be at home by themselves and to have a social group whom they could talk to and network with. After two years of working with them, we realized that they were our best ambassadors for the programs that we were opening at the Family Resource Center (FRC) because in our Latino cultures, the elders, their voices are very powerful. So we invited the Quinceaneras to help us do outreach for our FRC events and programs. As the Center Supervisor, I could make a bunch of calls, but I could never reach as many families as one of these women who has been in our community for 20 years. The voices of the Quinceaneras are very respected. It's a

wonderful, wonderful group. They bring food and have conversations between themselves and with the children and families in our program. And now they have started dancing Folklorico for the children in our program and for the larger community. As a result of participating in the Quinceaneras, their self-esteem has grown so much that they are now presenting for schools. In fact, last year they were dancing at Christmas in the park downtown.

(Rosalie Estrada, Family Resource Center Supervisor, Educare in Silicon Valley, San Jose)

◆ **Building a healthy identity and a sense of belonging.** Resilience is strengthened when children and adults are supported to build healthy identities rooted in their cultural ways of knowing and being and when they feel a sense of belonging.

◆ **Connecting families to community supports and resources.** Whether you have a small family childcare home or you work within a larger program/organization, preparing a list of resources you can share with families when in times of need, is foundational. Being able to provide or connect families to services or resources that can help to meet their physical, emotional, financial or basic survival needs will support them in building resilience and healing. As Rosalie Estrada, Supervisor for a Catholic Charities Family Resource Center, explains, it is important to let families lead the way in identifying their needs and requesting support.

'**Focus on building relationships first"**—Rosalie Estrada, Family Resource Center Supervisor, Catholic Charities

Our approach is to build a relationship with families first, and then later, when we are having a conversation and they express they're interested in or need something, that's when we connect them to services, classes or community resources. I think it is essential that I never make the parents feel that they are failing. I would never tell them, "you need to enroll in this service or take this child development class." In fact, at first, we don't even mention the classes we offer; we just introduce ourselves and give them a tour of the Family Resource Center. Our focus is on making a connection with the families. The next time I see them, I might mention that we have a class that is wonderful; parents like it because it provides them with just a little bit of extra support, and it creates an opportunity for them to network with other parents. I think that helps the parents to receive what I'm saying in a more positive way, "She's not telling me I'm a bad parent. She's just telling me I can learn something and meet some other families by joining this class." And I think that makes a huge difference.

Telling a family what they need or what they should do always has an undertone of "you are not good enough" and will be triggering emotionally for them. Within a context of a trusting relationship, we all become more open to hearing and exploring new ideas that may propel us to choose a new path toward learning, strengthening resilience and healing. In the next vignette, Valendena Koneck-Wilcox, a Family Engagement Specialist in Omaha, Nebraska, describes her agency's approach to connecting parents and families with community resources, especially mental health supports:

We connect families to all different types of community resources: The food pantry, free clothing and **a lot of my referrals are for mental health supports** which usually takes many conversations as there can initially be a lot of resistance for mental health services. Often times I'm teaming up with the teacher or others who are involved including the mental health consultant who works on site with our children. We work as a team to support a parent to connect with mental health supports. A lot of times we make the phone call together. Even so, we might make a phone call, set up an appointment and then they don't go. So it's an ongoing process. Until recently we had a mental health consultant here on site that was available for staff as well as parents. Having her on site was really helpful as she created a bridge to services. It can feel like a big leap for a parent to make a phone call, set up an appointment and go to a new place on their own.

(Valendena Koneck-Wilcox, Family Engagement
Specialist, Educare, Omaha)

Drew Giles, Director of Educator Programs, Franklin-McKinley School District at Educare, Silicon Valley connects with community partners in order to support his staff to gain the skills and to have the support they need to work with parents and families impacted by trauma. He explains:

Our Family Resource Center team is working with **Capacitar** (https://capacitar.org/). It is a healing-based organization. Our staff has worked with them for years to get support in developing skills on how to talk with parents and support the families who are going through difficult situations. Our classroom staff have also been working with Rebekah's Children's Services with their mental health specialists who are coming to our monthly meetings or as needed, when the staff feels like they want additional support, just to have someone to talk to. It's free, confidential and it helps them with their mental wellbeing. I didn't initially know how much my team needed that outlet to process. Because we care so much, we tend to not give our own problems the importance that they need. None of us realized how much we were taking in until we got the Capacitar training. The training helped us think about how to support families who are going through trauma. How to validate what they're going through and learn to recognize that something may be very simple for me, but because I don't know a family's situation and whole history, we never know how heavy an issue may be for a family. So never minimize their challenges.

The Importance of Inter/Intra-Agency Collaboration in Family Engagement

María Sujo, Kindergarten Readiness Program Manager, in a large urban school district, shares how inter-agency collaboration is the key to their ability to engage with culturally and linguistically diverse families and to break down systemic inequities many marginalized families face in the public school system. María explains how her office partners with teachers and cross-disciplinary community agencies to increase access for families to successfully enroll their children for kindergarten:

> We consider Kindergarten Readiness to be the work of the community, schools and adults to create the conditions for children to succeed. Some families of young children in our district, namely those furthest from opportunity, often struggle with a multi-step digital enrollment process that occurs one year before the start of kindergarten. We see the results of this hardship when children do not show up to the first day of school or are enrolled weeks later causing disruptions to their learning.
>
> COVID-19 exasperated this issue as schools are closed, making it harder to connect with families. So we partnered with the student enrollment unit, translations services, the Oakland Housing Authority, public health and kindergarten teachers to provide enrollment information sessions. We explained the enrollment process to families, provided health information and an opportunity to meet kindergarten teachers. Our relationships with the various city agencies are the glue that helps us connect and serve thousands of families of young children. A similar and more individualized process was used for our preschool families receiving special education services, due to their individual needs.

Though many of our families have a history of being marginalized by the education system, our relationship-based work and commitment to equity is helping us re-write the script, as to how families are received in our schools. We are creating a space where families are valued and can be in conversion with school and community leaders and can efficiently access the support they need to thrive.

(María Sujo, Kindergarten Readiness Program Manager, Early Childhood Education, Oakland Unified School District)

◆ **Perceiving a sense of agency and control.** As a loss of control is one of the conditions of a traumatic experience, gaining a felt sense of agency—i.e., having a voice and feelings of control is essential for coping and healing from trauma. When we provide opportunities for families to make choices, to influence programming, or provide input and feedback and elevate their voice, we are creating the conditions that helps people to heal from trauma and adversity.

In the following vignette, we see Chantelle Marin, a lead preschool teacher in Nebraska, applying this trauma-responsive practice in her work with families. Chantelle is knowledgeable about the neurobiology of stress and trauma and she regularly implements trauma-responsive practices. She understands that when a terrible thing happens within a family, especially to a young child, acknowledging the trauma and supporting the family to grieve and process their pain is important. You will see in her story how she responded to the tragic death of a child in her class using a trauma-responsive approach.

We had a family where over a weekend, one of the children in my class was in a bad car accident and actually passed away. That was very difficult for not only us as teachers, but also for the families of the students in my room. We were together with this child for multiple years and so it was really hard on all of us. Knowing that I had to come back and tell these little kids that their friend wasn't going to be there anymore, that was really difficult, especially at their age. I had a lot of conversations with all of the families in my class-room. For the grieving parents, I took their cues about what they wanted me to share or not share about what happened. With the other parents, I asked each one of them, "How do you want me to address this with your child?" Every family shared the language they were going to use to explain it to their child ("he is up in the clouds"). For a while afterward, I observed that a lot of the children's story dictation and their play included connections to this child's death. It was a way for them to make sense of it and to work through it. By honoring that and writing down their words or supporting them to include this theme in their play, we were letting the children and families know that we were there to support them; we were willing to listen to them and that we cared about them. I wanted not only the adults to have feelings of agency and voice in this traumatic situation; it was also really important to our teaching team that the children had a voice and that they knew we were listening to them.

Chantelle offered her classroom families opportunities to process and cope with this tragedy. She created opportunities to listen and attune to them and be responsive to their needs and choices (e.g., identifying the language and framing they preferred in talking about death with their young children; supporting the children to work through their fears and feelings in expressive art, dictation and play). She frequently checked in with the grieving family to show how much she cared and to listen to how they wanted her to share the news within the classroom and the larger school community. Chantelle was very intentional about giving all those whose lives were touched by this traumatic event a voice and opportunities for agency. It is common to have the urge to want to swoop in and begin to direct, tell, fix or offer solutions because we feel like we need to do something to be helpful. But being trauma-responsive is holding a safe space for people by listening and attuning to them and offering support through a caring relationship.

Applying the Trauma-Responsive Family Engagement Principles to the Language in an Early Childhood Program's Parent Handbook

Language is powerful. The words we choose to use send important messages to parents and families we engage with on a daily basis. Below, we share several examples that highlight how language—in this case within a parent handbook—can be adjusted to better reflect the goals and values of a trauma-responsive approach.

The examples in the right-hand column are not in any way intended to represent universal "best practice" recommendations. As discussed throughout this book, we believe that language used in early learning programs needs to be culturally, linguistically and individually responsive to the specific program philosophy, the children and families being served and the community context. Instead, we offer these as examples to inspire readers to consider how you can make adjustments in the language you use when communicating with families to reinforce the ideas embedded in the trauma-responsive principles discussed throughout this book (e.g., trusting relationships and partnerships, safety and predictability, strengths and assets, agency and control, disrupting inequity, cultural and linguistic diversity and strengthening resilience and healing).

Instead of this	*Try this*
Clothing for school Children should be dressed in comfortable play clothing, Play and learning activities often involve paint, water, clay and glue, which often end up on children's clothing. Dress your child for easy toileting. Clothes that are simple and washable are most appropriate. Overalls, leotards and belts are difficult to remove and contribute to accidents. Well-fitted shoes with flexible soles, such as tennis or running shoes are best; poorly fitted shoes can cause accidents.	**Clothing for school** We strive to make sure children can feel safe, engaged and to maximize their learning experience. We encourage clothing that allows for children to play easily and have fun. Because we play in dirt, with paint, water, clay and glue, their clothing may get dirty during the day. It is recommended to dress your kids for activities such as running, swinging, dancing, spinning, art, climbing, sand play, etc. If you need ideas, have concerns or need resources accessing this type of clothing, contact us at 1-800-555-5555 and our family engagement specialists will connect you to resources for clothing, or speak with you about any questions or concerns you have regarding these recommendations. We see you as a partner with us in the care and education of your child. We are here to listen and learn from you about what is best for your child and family.

Trauma-Responsive Principles Reflected in the Revised Language

Provide Opportunities for Agency and Control—The "after" conveys more of a sense that if parents have concerns, they can have a voice and are invited to provide input, or to make choices, that best fit the needs of their child. When policies are written in language such as "children should…" or "this is the rule " it takes away the family's voice and the requirement can often trigger stress reactions.

Create Power-Sharing Partnerships—The "after" conveys more of a bi-directional approach, a collaboration or reciprocity and moves away from the "dominant" stance in the first one which conveys "do as we say." In using humility in the language we use, we can approach families with respect and openness to challenge policies or procedures that may not fit within their needs, culture, values or perceptions.

Instead of this	Try this
Marking clothing Please mark all clothing with a permanent marker, ink or a label. We cannot take responsibility for unmarked clothing lost at the center. Preschool children need to keep one change of clothes in their cubby. Please ensure their cubby always has their change of clothes.	**Marking clothing** We recommend marking all clothing with permanent marker or labels so that your child's clothing will be safe and reduce the chances of another child accidently taking it home or it getting lost. When you arrive at the center, teachers will ask you if they can mark your child's clothing. Alternatively, you can mark or label your clothing if you prefer from home. Should you have any concerns about marking clothing please let us know. Teachers will not mark clothing without your permission.

Trauma-Responsive Principles Reflected in the Revised Language

Understanding Stress and Trauma and Provide Opportunity for Agency and Control—When families have cumulative stress factors, it may mean they cannot access their cortex. Therefore, too many instructions that involve one-way (you do the following) can be overwhelming to families. Rewriting a policy as shown above, conveys clear expectations but cultivates options for families, "we can do this together, or you can choose to do it at home, and you have a voice to let us know if you do not want certain clothing marked." It also communicates that we may not have considered all of the factors that influence whether this is a workable request for your family...in other words, it leaves open that we can learn from families and it conveys a sense of humility that communicates a message that it is safe to approach the staff with new ideas.

Instead of this	Try this
Nutrition program Our central kitchen prepares all snacks and meals daily for your children. All meals meet or exceed limitations of fat, sodium, saturated fat, calories, additives/ dyes, trans fats required by the law.	**Nutrition program** Our kitchen cares about the health and wellbeing of your child. They prepare home-made meals with love and that follow all the recommendations of My Healthy Plate (www.choosemyplate.gov/). However, we know every child has unique dietary needs or allergies. Please let us know at enrollment or by calling this number (1-800-555-5555) so that we may discuss this further and come up with a plan/solution that will work for you and your child.

Trauma-Responsive Principles Reflected in the Revised Language

Implement Culturally, Linguistically and Contextually Responsive Practices—The "after" recognizes that families come from cultural backgrounds that may have specific dietary needs, restrictions or limitations and creates an environment that recognizes, honors and allows for the different values and beliefs around food practices, preparation or dietary expectations.

Establish Safety and Predictability—In the after, we convey that we care about your child's health and wellness and can create safe and predictable environments by providing for their basic needs of food and nutrition AND that they can be individualized based on the dietary limitations your child may have.

Instead of this	Try this
Open-door policy Our program's open-door policy is in effect and parents are always welcome during our hours of operation. In the event a parent or guardian wishes to speak to a teacher directly, a mutually agreed upon time will be established for the conference.	**Open-door policy** There are multiple ways in which families can connect with teachers or administrators. We always want to make sure our parents and families are comfortable sharing their input, suggestions, feedback and concerns. Here are some of the ways you can talk to one of our team members in the agency: 1. Check-in daily with your teacher 2. Request a formal meeting 3. Complete the quarterly survey we mail out to families in multiple languages 4. Leave feedback in the suggestion box 5. Call us at 1-888-555-5555 and our office assistant will connect you to someone who can listen and help 6. Speak with the Family Liaison who is an advocate for all parents and families in the program 7. If you have additional suggestions, we are open to hearing them.

Trauma-Responsive Principles Reflected in the Revised Language

Use Culturally, Linguistically and Individually Responsive Practices. The "before" does not convey that there are multiple ways to communicate a concern. The language establishes that the open-door policy follows one pathway; a formal and mutually agreed upon time for a formal conference. It eliminates alternative pathways to communicate informally (drop in and chat), privately (confidential surveys, email, suggestion box), in writing (formal surveys), or through family meetings and gatherings. Additionally, the before option does not create pathways of communication in the language the family feels most comfortable with. Some families feel safer communicating a concern through a neutral person such as a family ombudsperson or liaison or in a private survey.

Establish Safety and Predictability and Provide Opportunities for Agency and Control. The before example states "open door" but actually appears to be one door only and that is through a formally scheduled conference. To move to a more trauma-responsive approach, the "after" signifies that we offer multiple open doors, not just one. By forming many pathways to communicate, we create a feeling of safety and predictability and families have more options to choose from that will align with their levels of comfort. For those who experience trauma, not having choices can trigger past memories of trauma when they felt out of control and had no options to protect themselves in duress. Further, when written policies or procedures are non-existent or ambiguous and unclear, it can lead parents and families to feel unsafe.

The "after" offers multiple ways of communication and ends with a final one that includes the idea that "we may have missed one that works better for you. You tell us what works for you."

Reflection/Discussion Questions

♦ If you work for a program with a family handbook, choose one policy, procedure or norm listed in the handbook. Thinking of the language used, are there changes you would make to make it more trauma-responsive?

References

Perry, B. (2017). *The boy who was raised as a dog and other stories from a child psychiatrist's notebook. What traumatized children can teach us about loss, love and healing.* New York, NY: Basic Books.

U.S. Department of Health and Human Services, Administration for Children and Families, Office of Head Start, National Center on Parent, Family, and Community Engagement. (USDHHS) (2018). *Key indicators of high-quality family engagement for quality rating Improvement systems*. Retrieved from https://childcareta.acf.hhs.gov/sites/default/files/public/indicators-final-508.pdf.

9

Father Engagement: Intentionally Planning for and Centering Fathers and Father Figures in Early Childhood

Historically, when we talk about family engagement, it's been about engaging mom and child. So when I think about family engagement, my first question is what are you doing to reach out to dad? What are you doing to ensure that dad has what he needs to be the best parent and the most active parent that he can be?

(Kevin Bremmond, Co-Founder and Program Administrator, Father Corps)

Over the last few decades, men's roles in their families and specifically, their interactions with their children have changed steadily. It has become increasingly common for men to stay at home with their children as the primary caregiver and for all fathers to participate more significantly in child rearing. However, there has not been an equal opportunity for men to have specific supports and training, a discovery Eric Peterson, Director of Client Services and Public Policy at BANANAS resource and referral agency, made 19 years ago when he found

DOI: 10.4324/9781003127666-10

out he was having a child. When Eric started attending a father support group he realized there was a significant unmet need for engaging fathers in his community: The first group only had four men enrolled and subsequent groups all had fewer than five men participating. In response to this experience, Eric has been supporting father engagement by leading father support groups in early childhood for 19 years. The groups are designed to support fathers and father figures to:

◆ Value their roles and needs as fathers
◆ Have opportunities to explore their thoughts, feelings and ideas about being dads with one another
◆ Provide support to one another
◆ Teach and learn together through listening, discussion, reflection and interactive experiences about rituals, rules, discipline, relationships and love
◆ Strengthen understanding of the needs of their children and if applicable, partners
◆ Improve their skills/ability to manage time, money, relationships, and expectations as fathers
◆ Have fun in community with other fathers

The monthly meetings address a range of topics including but not limited to different types and roles of fathers and father figures, the emotions associated with finding out you are going to be a father (e.g., joy, shock, denial/disbelief, acceptance...it's a process), transitioning into fatherhood, post-partum depression for men (and women), how to stay connected with kids, partner, friends and family while parenting and media portrayals of fathers. In these groups, fathers build connections with one another and learn about their thoughts, feelings and desires about being a dad through conversations and activities that ask them to explore:

◆ How they define what a father is (including a "good" father) and their personal beliefs about why fathers are important

- The rituals they had growing up that they want to carry forward and why they are important/meaningful to them
- How they want to prioritize their use of time
- Men they looked up to as a boy and what they admired in them
- Their beliefs, experiences, concerns and questions related to disciplining their child
- And then, during the final evening of class, the fathers explore two very emotional questions: **What kind of father did you have? What kind of father will you become?**

Nearly all of the fathers fall under two categories in this final discussion. The first group of fathers fear they will not develop into the idealized version of their father: the hero, caretaker, money maker, problem solver, coach. They have feelings of failing their family, their children and ultimately, never becoming the father they want to be. They often set unrealistic expectations of what a father is. Eric guides the fathers to spend time naming and working through these feelings together with the support of all of the other fathers. The other group of fathers is worried that they will become their fathers, the father that was not present, was abusive and drug and or alcohol addicted. These fathers are working hard to remove the ghosts that follow them. All of these men want the same thing: they want their children and partners to feel safe, free from trauma, to have a sense of freedom to be creative and to feel connected. Both of these groups of fathers express that they want their children to look back fondly at their childhood and have a sense of security and not fear that someday they will become great fathers.

Eric has discovered that although many of the men participate in his support groups because a spouse or partner signed them up, they find the experience to be really impactful and they continue to come throughout the entire series. And for many, they continue to maintain the relationships they build within the group for many years. Eric explains:

Before the class arrived I wrote 75 on the blackboard. After the men introduced themselves and broke into small groups to talk about the definition of what a father was, I asked each man how they ended up in class. I had discovered a pattern from previous groups. In every class at least 75% of the fathers are signed up by their partner. It was no different for this group and I told them that it was OK and many years of classes of fathers before them had the same reason for being here. I explained to them that the most important number was how many of them were going to be present for the last class. In all the years of teaching this class at least 90% of the fathers always made it to the end. The fathers I work with come from all income brackets, races, sexual orientations and philosophies. I often hear months and years later that many of these men made meaningful friendships and some of them continued meeting on their own after the class ended.

Eric recalls what it was like for Jorge, a new and young Latino father, when he first arrived in one of his fatherhood support groups:

Jorge was a new Latino father; he came into our 1st Fatherhood support group a few minutes late but just in time for introductions. He was a construction worker wearing his work gear and was dirty and had a metallic smell from the welding he had been doing all day. Jorge was stooped over and looked like he was in pain. He didn't look like the other fathers in our group; most of them were office workers, upper-middle class and White. Our classes are typically three to four– weeks long and the first two weeks we spend an extended amount of time in pairs having the fathers get to know each other in dyads. I have found that men don't typically open up in groups. Over the course of the first two weeks, the fathers all bond with each other and soon the similarities they have as fathers far outweigh their differences. Jorge became an important thought leader in the group. He shared with the fathers that he was initially apprehensive about having a child; their pregnancy was unplanned. He opened up that he personally had many problems and issues with his father while he was around.

A common theme among the men who have attended the support groups over the years is their relationships with their own fathers. Most fathers either live in fear of not being as good as their fathers or being as bad as their fathers. Jorge's father caused a lot of trauma in his family; he was physically and mentally abusive to Jorge's mother and Jorge. Each time Jorge attended the group, he was in a lot of pain. He had injured his back at work and believed he had to continue working to be "the man of the house." His wife was a successful Information Technology manager and had asked him to stay home and heal and spend time with their baby. Jorge shared this with the group and over the course of the 4 weeks of talking with the other fathers, he decided that it was the right decision to stay home. More importantly, the men all shared with Jorge and each other their common fears of becoming a good father. Two months after the group ended, Jorge called me and shared that he was nearly 100% physically healed and had decided to stay at home and care for his child for at least the next year. He thanked me and the group for the support and encouragement. Jorge has stayed in touch with several of the men in the group. He also started therapy to deal with the trauma from his childhood.

Fathers have very important roles in their children's life. Traditionally, fathers have felt they need to figure things out on their own. This can lead to isolation, uncertainty about their role and a lack of confidence in whether they are doing the right thing. When men gather in support, they have the opportunity to hear other struggles, ideas and solutions. They have a sounding board allowing them to talk about how they feel and to share their worries and concerns with one another. When this happens, it can reduce their feelings of isolation and sharpen their awareness of the range of feelings they have. Having opportunities to meet with other fathers can reduce stress as the relationships they build act as a buffer to stress and a source of support. Having opportunities to participate in groups like the fatherhood support groups Eric facilitates also create a time and space for men to pause and reflect on their aspirations, hopes and dreams for fatherhood so they can be intentional in their actions and parent in alignment with their expressed values.

Reflection/Discussion Questions

♦ What steps has your program taken to engage fathers? If you can take one additional next step, what might it be?
♦ What do you think the benefits would be for the families in your community if you were intentional about using father-engagement strategies? For fathers? For children? For families?

Another example of a program dedicated to centering the voices of fathers and father figures is **The Alameda County Fathers Corps**, a cross-sector collaborative formed to support fathers to be meaningfully engaged with their children and to advocate for father-friendly programs and services. The Father's Corps is staffed by a county-wide team of male service providers-in-training, who work to strengthen families by supporting men to be the best fathers they can be and to ensure their visibility within family serving organizations. The goal of the Fathers Corps is to ensure every father and father figure is fully engaged and supportive of their children and that agencies, schools and organizations are intentionally working to support fathers to succeed.

The Fathers Corps understands that children's development and educational resources and services are typically approached from a maternal perspective with the consequence that the needs and roles of fathers are often left out of programs and service delivery models for children and families. Further, because fathers are not intentionally thought about and planned for, many providers and agencies do not have the skills, knowledge and representation they need to effectively meet the evolving and diverse needs of fathers. To address these gaps and to support individuals and groups to intentionally plan for, and incorporate, fathers' needs into their programs and services, Father Corps developed several tools (free and downloadable from their website www. first5alameda.org/alameda-county-fathers-corps) that early childhood professionals can use to strengthen their Father Engagement Practices. These resources/tools are listed here and discussed in more detail below:

◆ Father-friendly principles
◆ Organizational self-assessment of father friendly services
◆ Father-friendly principles implementation tool, and
◆ The diversity of fathers photo bank

We developed father-friendly principles and an organizational self-assessment tool so organizations can assess how father friendly they are or not. Our implementation tool provides a step-by-step guide for organizations to implement each of the seven Father-Friendly Principles on a policy level, on a practice level, and on a staff level as well. We provide concrete, very practical activities that you can do to be more intentional and effective in engaging fathers.
(Kevin Bremmond, Co-Founder and Program
Administrator, Father Corps)

Alameda County Father Corps Seven Father-Friendly Principles for Agencies and Organizations

The Fathers Corps created the following seven Father-Friendly Principles that they recommend all agencies, programs and systems serving children and families integrate into their policies, procedures and practices:

Principle 1: Fathers and the needs of fathers, be included in the structure and delivery model of all family services

Principle 2: Programs, agencies and organizations be open, supportive, helpful and inclusive towards the needs of fathers and provide father-specific services and/or programs, all of which further the goal of increasing fathers' involvement in their children's lives

Principle 3: Outreach materials, illustrations, posters, brochures and other collateral materials include positive and diverse images of fathers being fathers, and that facilities provide father-friendly environments with materials consistent with the needs and interests of men and fathers

Principle 4: Family service programs, agencies and organizations create positions that serve fathers, and actively recruit men to fill those positions in order to better address the needs of fathers. To facilitate recruitment, we recommend development of a career track for father services, e.g., active recruitment of young men into social services with scholarships, internships and explicit advertising that "men are strongly urged to apply."

Principle 5: Programs, agencies and organizations working with families strive to provide training for all staff on working with men and on fatherhood issues

Principle 6: Programs, agencies and organizations develop program policies that include a clear expectation that fathers should and will participate

Principle 7: Programs, agencies and organizations make every effort to create the image that its programs are designed for fathers, as well as for mothers and children.

Find a link to the Principles here: www.first5alameda. org/files/Fathers_Corps/Alameda_County_Fathers_ Corps_-_Father_Friendly_Principles_Sheet.pdf.

Organizational Self-Assessment of Father-Friendly Services

The Fathers Corps designed an organizational self-assessment tool aligned with the seven Father-Friendly Principles to help individuals and groups assess their level of readiness to implement the Father-Friendly Principles and to identify both short-term and long-term action steps. The Organizational Self-Assessment Tool examines several areas of father-friendly practices:

- ◆ Assessing the needs of fathers
- ◆ Providing father-friendly services
- ◆ Using positive father images
- ◆ Creating positions that serve fathers
- ◆ Training staff on fatherhood issues
- ◆ Expecting father participation, and
- ◆ Designing programs for fathers

On the following page is a sample of the items on the Organizational Self-Assessment Tool. Users are encouraged to rate their program or agency's current practices versus what they aspire to be.

Include Needs of Fathers	Not Applicable (N/A)	Haven't thought about this or don't know	Started to think about this, but haven't made progress	Made good efforts, but have work to do	Efforts have been successful/ Ongoing progress expected
	0	1	2	3	4
1. All family services include a father-specific component.	☐	☐	☐	☐	☐
2. Parenting groups have been designed with both mothers' and fathers' issues in mind.	☐	☐	☐	☐	☐
3. Program hours accommodate the time constraints of working fathers.	☐	☐	☐	☐	☐
4. Organization's mission, vision, and/or value statements explicitly state the importance of including fathers.	☐	☐	☐	☐	☐

FIGURE 9.1
Organizational self-assessment
Source: Father Corps

Find the complete assessment tool here: www.first5alameda.
org/files/Fathers_Corps/Father-Friendliness_Organization_
Self-Assessment_REVISED_5.23.2017.pdf.

Father-Friendly Principles Implementation Tool

After completing the Organizational Self-Assessment, the Father-Friendly Principles Implementation Tool provides ideas on how to incorporate the Father-Friendly Principles into a program or organization's policies and practices. The implementation tool emphasizes *client and practice implementation* (e.g., to become father friendly in client interaction and service delivery to individuals, community groups, and families), *staff capacity building implementation* (e.g., building staff and leadership capacity to support organizational change to become father friendly) and *system and policy implementation*. Find the implementation tool here: www.first5alameda.org/files/Fathers_Corps/20182019/FatherFriendly_Principles_Implementation_Tool_19Sep18_Final.pdf.

The Diversity of Fathers Photo Bank

The Father Corps Diversity of Fathers Photo Bank includes a wide range of professional quality photos of diverse fathers and father figures with young children (www.diversityoffatherhood.com/). All of the photos are available for free download and use for non-profit organizations with an agreement that the photo credits will be given to the Father Corps. The photos reflect positive images of fathers and young children and there is an emphasis on images of Black fathers and fathers of color. The photo bank is a powerful example of strength-based images that disrupt stereotypes and deficit narratives about fatherhood.

One of the most powerful things that we can do to combat prejudice is really have more trust and connection and understanding and awareness as it relates to engaging families. Get to know us dads. We can tell within 30 seconds if you really give a damn about us so it can't just be lip service. Dads have to feel connected to someone and it's more than just words to establish that. Just like kids want and need to feel safe, parents need to feel safe. Parents need to feel like they're not judged, and that's for both moms and dads.

(Kevin Bremmond)

"**Being intentional in calling out fathers when you want them to participate is important**"—Kevin Bremmond, Co-Founder and Program Administrator, Father Corps

In the following vignette, Kevin Bremmond, Co-Founder of Father Corps, points out how important it is **to be intentional in planning to engage with fathers**. This includes considering the images you use to ensure that the diverse constellations and structures of families are represented. Also, to make an effort to be inclusive of fathers in the language chosen and the options for fathers to participate as well as learning from fathers by asking them what they want and need as partners in their child's early learning program. Kevin explains:

Programs, teachers, whomever, must extend invitations and build programming that supports fathers' needs. Instead of offering a parenting support group, try offering a father's support group. Instead of having a parenting night, have a dad's night. Historically, when we talk about parents, what we hear as dads is "mom" a lot of times because those services have historically been geared towards moms. So **being intentional in calling out fathers when you want them to participate is important.** If you're having a parent night consider the images that you use on materials advertising the event. Does it indicate that you want dads to show up? Are the images of dad and child? Usually it's a mom and child. Be specific with the language; include fathers in the wording because even when a provider says parent, subconsciously, many dads aren't thinking about themselves, we think mom. Consistency is also important; not just calling dad when you need the fence fixed at the school or the garden built, or to man the barbecue at the school cookout. Bring them in and ask them what they need. And know that families are different. Some families co-parent and don't live together so have awareness of the needs of the family and child being in two different households and that the two parents may not have the best communication. Go out of your way to make sure that you know each family's circumstances and the parental preferences for communication if possible.

Kevin also emphasizes the importance of not making assumptions about fathers and/or their roles in families and knowing that we need to both plan for their engagement but also identify their unique and individualized desires for participation. This begins by creating welcoming messages that are inclusive but also adopting a listening and learning stance to get to know each individual father and their child and family context in order to be responsive and learn about the ways they want to engage in the early learning program.

Reflection/Discussion Questions
- ◆ In what ways do you engage with fathers?
  - What about the language you use at intake, outreach, events, communication?
  - How do you advertise your parent engagement events to include fathers?
  - In what ways do you intentionally plan to include fathers?
  - How do you individualize parent engagement so as to not assume all fathers come from the same family constellation or have the same roles within families?
- ◆ Have you ever asked the fathers in your program what they need and how they would like to engage in the program's services?

Father Engagement: Fathers and Father Figures Want to Have Their Voices Heard

In the following vignette, Kevin Bremmond offers suggestions for engaging Black fathers in early childhood programs. He shares many strategies that strengthen father engagement for all fathers but especially for Black, Indigenous and Fathers of Color who have historically been the least likely to be included in parent involvement programs. As you read through this story, consider what you are already doing and what action steps you could work on to communicate to fathers that you are intentionally working to include them, make them feel welcome and to be responsive to their needs.

> We have to start off with the assumption that Black fathers want to be involved and if they are not involved, that they do want to be involved. I think a lot of times we start from the opposite direction and we assume that dads aren't involved and that they don't want to be. And then there's the simple things. Say hello. Don't ignore us. Be authentic with your engagement. Don't over celebrate when you see a Black dad with their kids like it's an anomaly or something. Just give Black dads the same grace you give everyone else. We're not the only ones who have families that look different. The idea that families have to be married, you know, with three kids and a White picket fence, this is not how families look. So let's not be judgmental about divorced, separated, single or co-parents. We need to normalize healthy co-parenting relationships because a lot of times what happens is mom is going to get services from one organization. And, you know, she could be on the outs with dad. If the mom is talking with the provider and then they both are now on the outs with dad, then we don't make progress. Just because the relationship with mom and dad doesn't work, that doesn't mean he needs to be left out of his kid's life. And I think as providers, a lot of times we jump on that train. A lot of

times dads feel like they are going at this thing alone and they don't have any real place to turn when it's their day or time with their child.

Using father-specific language is important. You know, I was a 19-year-old parent when I had my first child. And I can't say I would have gone to something at my child's preschool at 19 but I remember being invited to a playgroup and I had no idea what that was. I was 19 and I wasn't going to go to a play group. I'm too cool for that. So I think language is important from a cultural standpoint but also an intergenerational standpoint. Programs have to be creative you know and talk to the dads themselves. Find out their needs, likes or dislikes. Let them name your program. Find out what your dads are into and go that direction. Let them lead. Men know what their kids need, want and what their kids like. They know what play looks like with their kids. Let's follow their lead instead of us telling them what they should be doing. You need men who are running some of these programs. Men need to be in the front of the room. Whatever it is that you're offering, it's a lot easier for men to connect with other men which can be hard as a lot of social and family support services are staffed by a majority of women.

Surveys can be a good way to get information from dads because information gathering can be done outside of a conversation. Also, incentives are important or a good way to engage dads, if programs can afford them. If you gotta give us a $25 gift card or a $50 gift card to get us through the door, then that's what you gotta do. And then you have to offer a program that's compelling enough that we will come back when you are no longer offering that incentive. If you're an organization that his-torically has not served dads, it's gonna take you some time to get dads to trust you, to understand that the program is built for them and for them to show up and come back. Father engagement has to be supported—leadership has to be bought in. It's important for funders to understand this as well. If you're a new organization serving dads for the first time…our numbers might not be what we want them to be during the first couple of months or couple of quarters, you (funders) have to give us some time to build that trust and build those relationships.

Review the father-engagement strategies in the vignette above and identify your strengths (what you are already doing) and your learning edges (what you want to work on implementing):

◆ Reflect on your mindset: Are you assuming all fathers want to be involved, especially our Black, Indigenous and Fathers of Color?

◆ How do you greet fathers every day when they arrive/pick up their children?

◆ Do you act surprised or "over celebrate" when dads, especially Black dads, are engaged with their children and your program?

◆ How do you acknowledge and respect diverse family structures and plan to support co-parenting relationships in ways that ensure that fathers are included (e.g., services, communication, etc.)?

◆ When do you use father-specific language?

◆ In what formats do you ask dads about their interests, needs and goals related to parenting? Do you listen to what they say and integrate their ideas into the program?

◆ Have you created opportunities for dads to have agency and control—voice and choice—in family engagement formats and activities? Do you support fathers to have leadership and be "in front of the room"?

◆ Offering incentives for dads' involvement may be a way to outreach to fathers and engage them. Is this something your program has thought about or is able to do? If not, what are other incentives or outreach strategies that you can think of?

◆ List opportunities you provide for dads to be engaged or ideas you have for the future to engage with fathers?

◆ Is there support and "buy in" from your program/agency leadership to support father engagement?

◆ How do you build trust with fathers? Given historical patterns of marginalizing fathers, is there an explicit acknowledgment that timelines and outcomes must be realistic and awareness that building trust will take time?

10

Case Studies: Applying Ideas throughout the Book to Your Practice

♦ **Case Study #1: "What Positives Have You Noticed About Your Own Daughter at Home?"**

A Trauma-Responsive Approach to Communication with Parents Going through a Conflictual Divorce—Svetlana Popov, Kindergarten Teacher, Ashland School District

Danika and Charlie are living in different apartments and are going through a challenging and conflictual divorce. When married they fought frequently in front of the children. Now that they are separated, they refuse to speak with one another and can't agree on any terms for visitation or common ways to raise their children. They accuse the other of poor parenting and align with the children against the other parent. They have three children, one enrolled in kindergarten, one in 3rd and another in 5th grade at John Middleton public elementary school. The youngest, 6-year-old Katrina is regressing (having accidents at school,

DOI: 10.4324/9781003127666-11

frequent tantrums at drop-off, verbally fighting with other children) and the other parents are complaining to the principal that this child is a problem who needs to be removed from the classroom. Her parents are difficult to reach and blame the other parent for the child's behavioral challenges. Katrina's kindergarten teacher, Svetlana Ivanov has tried to engage Katrina's parents individually about their daughter's challenges but every conversation turns into blaming the other parent. The parents refuse to be in the same room with each other and say meeting together is out of the question.

After consulting with her principal, Malcolm Price, Teacher Svetlana agreed to a plan and to move forward with specific next steps. She worked with Principal Price to provide trauma-responsive strategies in the classroom so that Katrina felt safe, had a predictable routine and nurturing connections. Teacher Svetlana looked below the surface of the challenging behaviors and found strategies to reduce opportunities for Katrina to become dysregulated by increasing supports for her during the times that most seemed to trigger her such as drop-off time and when she is in the bathroom. Drop-off time is an especially triggering transition for Katrina, so Teacher Svetlana created a routine that helped Katrina reduce the abruptness and allow her to slowly warm up to the transition and start of her day. She would welcome Katrina each morning when she arrived and spend time connecting with her more intentionally to help her make a less abrupt transition into the classroom. She would greet her and ask how she was feeling, "Good morning Katrina. Would you like to check-in this morning with our feeling chart? I can put my name on what I feel and then you can too. Would you like to go first or do you prefer that I start?" She invited Katrina to use the "calm zone" if she indicated her feelings were dysregulated and if she felt that would help her. Svetlana had a special calming corner in her room. In the calming corner, she had sensory materials such as art supplies, books about feelings and breathing ideas, nature posters, bubbles for breathing and a regulation poster the kids put together with ideas for calming their bodies. Katrina often chose to use this space when invited for a slow transition into the classroom and until she was ready to start her day. Teacher Svetlana knew that starting with small steps to help Katrina feel safe and stay regulated was a top priority.

After talking with her principal, Teacher Svetlana realized that she was triggered by Katrina's parents' behavior and these feelings were preventing her from being intentional in her responses with them. She discovered that she was "soaking in" their anger and finding herself being pulled down into their dysregulated state (e.g., as she imagined herself demanding that they come into the school where she would command them to stop acting this way and lecture them about how they were both harming their children). Being able to talk about her frustrations and big emotions with her principal allowed her to de-escalate, return to a regulated state and brainstorm how she could restore her energy when she was feeling stressed or burned out so she would have the emotional reserves to keep her own cortex (thinking and problem solving) engaged. Together with her principal, she made her list: Outside of work she would take short walks, cook, talk with friends and eat healthy meals. While she was at work, her principal would support staff self-care by providing what he called a "touch and go self-care system." Anytime a teacher needed a short break, they could use their classroom phone to press 1426 which went directly to the counselor's office. All the teachers had to say is, "can I get a temporary sub to use the restroom" or "can I get a sub for a brief moment." This self-care strategy is used when teachers need a brief momentary break to regroup.

Teacher Svetlana took these small steps in her work with Katrina and found that she responded very positively to them. She was intentional in sharing small daily success stories with each of Katrina's parents at pick up. She acknowledged Katrina's positive attributes and strengths in a manner that reduced the stress levels for each parent and promoted a positive connection between parent/child at pickup. For example, she might say, "You must be doing something right as a parent because Katrina has such a kind spirit...here is an example of what she did today to show such kindness..." As she began to share positive observations, she found herself building more of a positive connection with each of Katrina's parents. Sharing these successful moments was intentional for Svetlana: She hoped that each parent would begin to shift their internal state of stress toward thinking of the well-being of their daughter. She also shared with them these positive attributes about their daughter to build the parent-child connection. Finally, she used this strategy because the parents' focus was continually on their own internal stress states and they often forgot to see Katrina and that she needed them to attune and connect with her to help buffer her stress. Teacher Svetlana began to slowly ask each parent a simple question—**what positives have you noticed about your own daughter at home?** Are they similar to what I am observing at school? Over time, she shifted from a focus on what she observed as Katrina's strengths at school, to guiding Katrina's parents to focus on and name what they experienced/observed as their daughter's strengths and positive attributes. It took a few months, but Teacher Svetlana noticed a significant shift in her interactions with Katrina's parents. Communication shifted from complaining about the other parent or defensiveness about Katrina's behavior towards seeing strengths and connecting with their daughter.

What Trauma-Responsive Family Engagement Core Principles Are Seen in This Case Study?

Principle: Understanding Stress and Trauma. Most teachers might take the fastest route by looking at, and reacting to, the surface of the presenting behaviors. Trauma-responsive family engagement is not always the fastest and most obvious path. When early childhood professionals are triggered, it would be easy to become reactive to the challenging behaviors of the adults and/or child and react with threats of punishment, directives, expulsion or exclusionary practices for Katrina and/ or her parents. Such quick fix strategies use power and threats ("Do as I say or we can no longer serve your child in this program") and can bring fast results but can also be trauma-inducing, adversely impacting all relationships and cause a longer-term distrust and disruption in the family's ability to trust others in authority or the system. It is difficult to have 20 or more kids in a classroom with one or more children who has intensive challenges. When we understand that stress or traumatic experiences can disrupt both children's and adults' sense of safety and their ability to access their cortex (thinking, problem solving, regulation), then educators can do what Teacher Svetlana did which is not to personalize the behavior and not to see it as intentional or frame it as bad. Understanding stress and trauma also means cultivating self-awareness of our own triggers. Teacher Svetlana—with the support of her principal—came to recognize the signals of stress in her body. Her principal helped her understand that if she did not take care of her stress, she might default to reactive behavior (fight, flight or freeze) that could cause further harm. By building her self-awareness and working with her principal to identify several trauma-responsive strategies she could implement right away, she was supported to manage her own internal state of stress in emotional emergencies.

Reflection/Discussion Questions

- ◆ Can you think of a child/family who presented with challenges that you have worked with? How have you used supervision as a way to express and vent built-up emotions so that you could begin to calm and plan for responsive strategies that would help the child/family?
- • How do you implement self-care or restorative strategies outside of work so that when you arrive in the morning,

you have the energy reserves to cope with challenges (work, child, family, colleagues) without becoming reactive?

◆ Does your program intentionally promote any self-care strategies or support services that promote self-awareness, health, wellness and/or self-care?

Principle: Establish Safety and Predictability. Family engagement practices can begin where we, as early childhood educators, create for children and/or families a feeling of being safe, having a predictable routine and relational connections that are nurturing. In this case study, it is starting with, and prioritizing, the well-being of Katrina. Providing Katrina with a safe and predictable environment and a nurturing, responsive relationship were essential. And, for the teacher to reinforce feelings of safety for Katrina and to give her activated stress responsive system some reprieve. Teacher Svetlana was determined to work with her principal on ways she could utilize trauma-responsive strategies to support Katrina during this time of traumatic stress. She created a ritual at drop-off that recognized the abrupt transition from home to school was a pain point where Katrina was becoming triggered. When Katrina arrived at school, she was highly stressed. Finding a temporary ritual where Katrina could arrive, be by herself in the classroom calming corner and to engage when she was ready, seemed to work well during the morning transition. Teacher Svetlana also increased the dosage of personal and positive interactions—relational pathways to regulation—with Svetlana at drop-off and throughout the day to help her maintain feelings of safety and calm. Simple acts of kindness such as sharing a private positive comment ("You are so helpful"), a brief dose of a personalized check-in (going up to Katrina and sitting down and chatting with her), allowing Katrina to sit close to her during circle time, and/or providing extra support during challenging assignments were all intentional actions Teacher Svetlana took to help Katrina have a felt sense of safety at school.

Reflection/Discussion Questions

◆ Can you think of a child who is frequently dysregulated that you have worked with and how you provided one or more of the following trauma-responsive strategies to create a safe and predictable environment (safe space, ritual around transitions, regulatory activities that calm activated stress such as emotional check-in charts)? A nurturing and responsive relationship that built a sense of safety and trust for the child (small moments of intentional connection or regulatory support)?

Principle: Focus on Strengths and Assets. Family engagement practices are rooted in using a strength-based approach that centers attention on the strengths, creativity/creative problem solving, sources of coping, resilience and well-being and potential in children and adults, families and communities. In this case study, Teacher Svetlana paused and asked herself "What is the point of entry?" to begin to connect with and engage one or both of Katrina's parents? She decided that the way to increase engagement and trust with the parents was to shift the conversations at drop-off or pick up to be about their daughter's strengths and positive attributes. Svetlana knew the parents were experiencing a lot of stress in their personal lives. She understood that asking them to focus on their daughter's challenges would only exacerbate their stress level and cause them to go more into avoiding her or to activating their stress response systems, so instead, she focused on building relational connections, trust and focusing on the strengths.

In this case, asking the parents about their daughter's strengths created small shifts in her relationship with the parents and moved the default conversation from blaming the other parent to their daughter and her well-being. The parents often got so caught up in their own emotions that they lost focus on their shared goal which is the well-being of their daughter. Helping them remember Katrina's well-being and supporting nurturing connections between the parent/child was an intentional and effective trauma-responsive family engagement strategy.

Reflection/Discussion Questions

◆ Have you experienced working with a parent or family where you were able to refocus the conversation on a shared goal or a strength as a point of entry into building a relational connection and improving trust and safety?

Think about a child and family you have worked with and found challenging for you in some way. Were there any trauma-responsive strategies you used and/or could have used?

◆ Were you able to observe the child over time and look past the dysregulated **surface** of the behavior to pause and look deeper at the meaning **behind** the child's behavior? Was the child's behavior communicating they felt unsafe (trauma related trigger), that they had big emotions (anger, sadness, disappointment, worry, happiness) or was the child's behavior communicating they needed someone or something?

◆ How did you start the conversation with the parent/s about their child's persistent dysregulated behavior? What was your point of entry? How did you feel doing this?

◆ Were you able to recognize your own stress levels and triggers around this behavior?

◆ In what ways did you manage your stress? Were there people that supported you within your workplace? Outside of your workplace? What activities help you restore your energy and buffer your activated stress response system? Are there organizational care routines in place that support staff to reduce their stress and feel supported?

◆ What other trauma-responsive strategies did you use in your interaction with the family/child?

◆ Case Study #2: "We Got This. Your Kids Are in a Safe Place All Day with Me"—Teacher Mariana, Owner, Hope Family Child Care Center

A single mother, Karyn and her two children Marcus (age 2) and Allison (age 4) are experiencing homelessness and temporarily living doubled-up in her friend Melissa's home. Karyn, with the help of her friend, packed up her kids while her partner was at work and moved in temporarily with Melissa after her partner started hitting and verbally threatening her. She has been living with Melissa for the past month and continues to work full time as a receptionist for a construction company. Karyn shares a bedroom with her two children. In another bedroom, is Melissa and her new boyfriend and there is one other family of four (two children ages 2 and 4) who are temporarily renting space in the garage due to a recent eviction from their apartment. All of them share one bathroom in the house.

Karyn and her children have been coming to Hope for Children, a small family child care for children birth to age 12 years for the past two years. Teacher Mariana (Owner) and Michael (her Teacher's Aide) are very caring to Karyn's children and her children have always loved attending Hope. The past few weeks, Karyn has been arriving late each morning and she has been avoiding interaction with teachers Mariana and Michael. Karyn's children show a new range of stress related behaviors. They are tired or fall asleep frequently throughout the day and have increased tantrums, whining and crying. Marcus tends to have frequent tantrums and his crying is persistent and inconsolable. Allison on the other hand, shows behaviors that are more regressive such as biting or throwing toys alternated by asking to be held and picked up. She won't let the teachers out of her sight and she becomes frightened if she cannot see them (e.g., when one of them goes to the bathroom). Marcus has become clingy and when strangers enter the child care home, he hides under the table. He refuses to nap and instead, wants

Mariana right next to him. Karyn and Teacher Mariana have always had a good connection but recently, Mariana has noticed that Karyn drops the children off and rushes back out of the door without her usual greeting, goodbyes and conversations. Karyn is often on her cell during drop-off and pickup avoiding any interaction with Mariana or Michael. Mariana is worried something is going on at home that may be causing these new behaviors from the children. She thought it would be helpful if she could talk to Karyn.

Today, Teacher Mariana welcomed Karyn at pick up time. She said to her, "You know how much I love your children and they mean so much to me. I wonder if we can find a few minutes to chat soon about the kids and some observations I am making." Karyn said she had to run out as she was late for something. She briskly prodded her kids to hurry up to get out of the door. The next morning, Mariana welcomed Karyn and her children and again she said:

> I know how much you care for your children. You are such a great mom. I am here to support you and the children. If you can find some time—even 15 minutes in your busy schedule to talk anytime day or night, I will make it happen. I am here to support you. We can also find child care for your kids if needed while we talk.

Teacher Mariana noticed that the tension in Karyn's face and shoulders softened hearing these words. Karyn took a deep breath in, let out a sigh and said she would think about it. Mariana said, "There is no pressure. We are here for you. We just want to continue to build on our positive connection and relationship for your children like we always have done in the past with one another."

That evening mom texted Mariana and said she was taking off work tomorrow. She asked, "Could we meet at 4:00 pm outside the center so the kids won't see me when I arrive?" Mariana said that of course this was fine and that she would meet mom outside on the front porch to chat. They met at 4pm the next day. Mariana started by offering mom a cup of tea or water and a snack of fresh baked cookies she made. Mom started to well up with tears. Mariana paused and took a deep breath reassuring Karyn, "It is okay, we are safe here together. There is privacy and if it is too much, you can take a break at any time. There is no hurry." Karyn's tears started pouring out and Mariana offered her a tissue. As Karyn wiped her eyes, she shared that this has been such a hard time. Her partner was being aggressive with her and it was happening in front of the kids. Karyn went on to say the verbal aggression was beginning to be directed to the kids and she was scared it would become physical next time. Karyn said she left home and is living with her friend temporarily in a small apartment. "I don't know where to go. The kids are having a hard time and are extra clingy with me and crying all the time and are not sleeping very well. I really don't know what to do next."

Mariana thanked mom for trusting her enough to share what was going on. She asked if she could give her a hug and then said, "**We got this together. Your kids are in a safe place all day with me.** We can tackle one thing at a time together." Mariana saw mom beginning to calm and feel a sense of relief and there was less tension in her face and her tone of voice was not as strained. Mariana prioritized mom's voice first by asking Karyn, "What is your most urgent need?" Karyn listed all the things she needed help with beginning with the most urgent—finding a place to live on her own. Mariana continued, "Do you feel safe in your current location? Do you feel like you are in any danger from your partner?" Karyn confirmed that she did feel safe at her friend Melissa's home. She was worried about her partner but to her knowledge, he did not know where they were staying. They discussed a safety plan (i.e., restraining order, emergency numbers for her to call, how the school will respond if he enters the school, communicating to the children in an age-appropriate way how they can stay safe). Next, was the impact on her children.

Mariana asked Karyn, "Do you want support connecting to community resources for help with housing, food, clothing, counseling or any other needs?" Karyn explained that she would like help identifying and contacting community services as she felt overwhelmed and had no family nearby to help her. Next, Karyn said she knew her kids were impacted by the whole situation but she personally felt too scared and overwhelmed to talk about it with them. Mariana asked Karyn if they could set up another time to talk so they could strategize together and how to support the kids. Karyn agreed and they decided to meet again in a few days. After finding out she felt safe and did not feel in eminent danger and that her basic needs such as food and clothing were being met, Mariana helped Karyn connect to their local early childhood resource and referral agency, the community helpline and local religious institutions so Karyn could begin to identify resources that could help her and her children. Mariana collected information about comprehensive community resources in an accessible file cabinet for families to access especially at difficult times like this. After having Mariana's support to connect with these community agencies, Karyn was able to sign up and qualify for counseling and add her name to a waitlist for housing services and to receive information about trauma-responsive strategies she could use to support her children during this time of uncertainty, stress and change.

What Trauma-Responsive Family Engagement Core Principles Are Seen in This Case Study?

Principle: Understanding Stress and Trauma. Mariana understood the impact of toxic stress on mom and her children. Even without knowing the history of what was happening, Mariana understood that all behavior is communicating something. She believed that Karyn's behavior was telling a story about the stress she was experiencing. If Mariana were to interpret the situation in her mind based on a surface-level understanding of Mom's behavior (an internal voice asking, *"What is wrong with you?"*) the cascade of behaviors she may have expressed to Karyn (short-tempered, threatening, critical and potentially shaming) would only make the situation worse. Instead, Mariana was able to pause and stay regulated so she could access her cortex and remember to move her internal voice to *"What is the meaning behind your behavior? What do you need to feel safe?"* With that internal voice, Mariana was able to employ a trauma-responsive approach to have empathy for Karyn, use a calm state to co-regulate Karyn's dysregulated state and guide her back to regulation by communicating in a nurturing and responsive manner and reinforcing messages of safety and security.

Reflection/Discussion Questions

♦ Have you ever been engaged in an interaction with a parent or family where you observed them having dysregulated behavior?

♦ Were you able to recognize your own internal reactions (internal voice, feelings, sensations, thoughts)?

♦ Do you have an example of when you paused, looked past the challenging behavior and tried to figure out the meaning of the behavior? Were there examples of how you pulled yourself back from a reaction that may have been trauma-inducing ("What is wrong with you?") to one that is more trauma-responsive ("What happened to you? What is your behavior communicating about what you need to feel safe"?)

Principles: Building Mutually Respectful and Trusting Relationships and Establishing Safety and Predictability. Teacher Mariana had spent two years building a relationship with Karyn and her children. This trusting connection allowed Karyn during this time of stress to feel a sense of safety with Mariana. Because they built a strong connection with one another, Karyn felt safe enough to share sensitive personal information with

Mariana and to seek her support and help. The routines and pre-dictability Mariana created for Karyn's children over the course of two years helped them create associations between Mariana's child care home and feelings of physical, social and emotional safety for their family. For example, at pick up time, Mariana had a daily routine of sharing one positive behavior or developmental milestone with Karyn about each of her children. This routine established a strong relational connection and communicated to the entire family, "You are significant, important and you belong here with us."

Reflection/Discussion Questions

◆ What are the strategies you use to intentionally build posi-tive relational connections with your families every day?

◆ Do you take steps to help families feel a sense of inclusion and belonging in your program? How do you do this?

◆ At drop-off and pick up, what specific strategies do you use with a parent or family to show you care and that your environment is safe for them and their children?

Principle: Provide Agency and Control. Knowing stress and trauma triggers leave people feeling fear and less in con-trol, Mariana made sure that she avoided language that would exacerbate these feelings for Karyn (e.g., "I am concerned about your children" or "We need to talk and it is urgent") and only further activate her stress response system. Instead, Mariana used trauma-responsive language such as "You are safe here." She offered Karyn choices—e.g., "We can meet when it is con-venient for you" or "We can take a break anytime you choose," giving Karyn opportunities to have control in their interactions. Mariana also focused on making sure Karyn was okay first before bringing up any concerns about her children. That kind of attunement to mom's emotional safety and well-being was regulating for Karyn allowing her to remember that she was in a safe place and to perceive that Mariana was a person who wanted to help her. *The words, the language and body cues we use convey messages to parents and families about whether they are safe and whether they have any power, agency or control in a situation.*

Reflection/Discussion Questions

◆ Did you notice any verbal cues that Mariana used to help convey safety and attuned connection with Karyn? Have you ever used these types of verbal cues that lead a family to regulation (calm) vs. dysregulation (distress)?

◆ Did you notice any nonverbal cues that Mariana used to help convey safety and attuned connections? Have you ever used these types of nonverbal cues that lead a family to regulation (calm) vs dysregulation (distress)?

◆ Thinking back on an interaction with a family that was stressful, were there any small ways you helped the family to feel they had a choice, input or a sense of agency and control in that moment?

◆ Case Study #3: "We Honor What You Bring to the Table"—Fela Barclift, Executive Director/Founder, Little Sun People

Fela Barclift is the Executive Director and the Founder of Little Sun People, an African-centric child care program in the Bedford Stuyvesant neighborhood of Brooklyn, New York serving children age 2 to age 5. She shares highlights of the approach to family engagement at Little Sun People:

> Parent Partnerships is one of our program's three foundational pillars. We want our welcome for parents to be deeply warm and sincere to communicate absolute respect for them. We really want parents to know that **you are essential here. And we care. We honor what you bring to the table.** Your relationship with your child is critical and we're never going to overstep that and act as if, just hand your child over. No, no, no, no! This is a partnership. We care about and respect you, and we welcome you with all the warmth and love that we have in our hearts. And you come in and stay as long as you need to including the parents of our 2-year-olds. They are invited to come in for an hour with

their child, stay with the child and visit the school, come to some of our celebrations, play in the park with us so that in September when they officially enter the program, the child already is a part of our community. That wrenching integration doesn't happen. Instead, it's a smooth slope. They can say goodbye without it turning into like a massive stress, you know. Who are these strangers? Some children can't wait for this new adventure and they're ready for their parents to go and to jump into the community. And then there's other children who are just terrified to let go. So we give them all the time they need for themselves and their parents to take their time and get to know us and feel safe here.

For a small Black school like ours, we have a powerful Parents Association. Our parents come out for our monthly meetings. I'm always invited to say a few words and to answer questions but the agenda is created and the meetings are led by our parents and we have a majority of the parents engaged in our Parents Association. We bring in the fathers. There are specific times when we have a very large fathers program. We document this because it's so important to the fathers, as well as to the children. We feel that people have talked so badly about Black dads—"They're not present in their child's life," "They don't know how to love." In our program, we highlight how dads do such an amazing job. We include dads throughout the program and have two times during the year when we specifically highlight our dads.

Parents practically live in this place! We can never get them out [laughing]. They are here every morning and come in the afternoons and evenings too. In mornings when they come in, they are visiting with each other and with the children. Any activity that our staff is trying to do, the parents are backing us fully. But our parents also initiate a number of things on their own. Parents make our yearbooks every year and this year, they created an amazing calendar. It was so beautiful! They made sure that we got everybody together for the pictures that they wanted to be included in the calendar. And they raised a little more than $15,000 for our school with a calendar event. They also plan experiences like a Paint and Sip event or a Roller-skating party. During Teacher Appreciation week our parents bring flowers, breakfast and gifts and show so much appreciation to our teachers. They're very, very supportive of the teachers' efforts and respectful towards them. At Little Sun People, we have many, many years of practice building a very strong parent engagement piece at our school.

I'm like the drum major for maintaining our focus on an African-centered perspective and over time it has become our program's culture. We have several really big, special events—ceremonies and celebrations— that we do during the course of the year and center our teaching around. For instance, during December we have our Kwanzaa celebration and there's so many things that are connected to the experience of celebrating Kwanzaa that teaches about African history, African culture, African values and valuing African people. These experiences help us to deeply connect with African culture. We also do a Black history celebration for a full month as well which gives us a chance to talk and think about many amazing people and the great things that they did. And we bring these messages to children in *their* language; in the language of a 2 year old or a 3 year old or 4 year old. "Look at these people. Aren't they amazing?" And they look just like you and your mommy and your daddy, your aunts and your uncles.

We also have a part of our school year when **we bring in the whole community**. We bring in everybody. We have aunties and uncles and cousins and nephews and nieces. Every child proudly brings forth this amazing adult that's connected to them. And they tell stories. They bring artifacts, and they bring their videos to share who they are and what their relationship is to this child. This is a proud moment for each young person and for us. We share stories of the present time as well as the ancient stories of our ancestors. And we bring it all together for the children and families at Little Sun People. The other stuff like teaching the alphabet and numbers and the colors and the shapes, we get that in the state standards. So the teachers can go through and integrate those things into their lessons. But, when they're planning and teaching, we consider, "What's the lens I'm using?" That's what we're constantly thinking about. Is the lens African centered? Does it connect to that child and his or her family and community? Or is it a generic lens that doesn't really connect to anything? It's just, "here's the facts, deal with it." All of our teachers are in growth and learning how to do this what we do. We don't have a model. We have to figure it out as we go. And that's what we're doing.

Fela Barclift and her staff are creating a program culture that embodies so many of the trauma-responsive principles discussed throughout this book. It is clear that they focus on families' strengths and assets. ("In our program, we highlight how dads do such an amazing job!") They are also very intentional about centering culturally, linguistically and community responsive practices that align with their families' diverse values, beliefs and practices. When Fela and her teachers plan curriculum or activities they ask themselves, "What's the lens I'm using? Is the lens African centered? Does it connect to that child and his or her family and community?" They support safety for children and families entering the program and center parents' voices and share power with them authentically allowing them to influence the program in many ways. And they create a sense of welcome whether intentionally planning for fathers or for children's diverse caregivers and families. Little Sun People creates a sense of belonging and community that supports children and adults to feel supported, cared for and visible.

Reflection/Discussion Questions

◆ How do you welcome each parent and family member in a manner that conveys the message "You belong, you are welcome, you are family, we care about you and your child"?

◆ How do you consider the cultural values, beliefs and practices of families and ask yourself "Will a child or family see themselves in my curriculum, activities, program and environment?"

◆ Case Study #4: "Ray's Parents Are from Europe and Maybe They Don't Understand What Appropriate Behavior Is"—Terry Marshall-Simmons, Site Supervisor, Pleasant Hill Child Development and Early Learning Center

Terry Marshall-Simmons is the Site Supervisor of the Pleasant Hill Child Development and Early Learning Center, a private center with children ages 3–5 and located in an urban community in Boston, MA. The teachers at this site are concerned about, Ray, a 5-year-old child, in one of the classrooms. Ray loves school and playing with his friends. He lives with mom, dad and 13-year-old brother in an apartment. His father works full time and mom stays home. There is no known history of trauma that anyone is aware of, however, when emotionally triggered, Ray threatens to harm his teachers. Alarmed by Ray's behavior, the teacher continually calls Ray's mother or father to pick him up following each of these incidents. The staff have repeatedly told their supervisor Terry and the regional director that they feel the other children are at risk and that Ray should be removed from the school. They report that they have tried everything to help Ray and nothing is working. They place the responsibility and blame on Ray's parents' shoulders saying, "Ray's parents are from Europe and maybe they don't understand what appropriate behavior is in our culture."

Terry and her staff have been attending a trauma-informed practices (TIP) training series provided by their agency for the past six months. Additionally, as TIP is a topic of tremendous interest to Terry, she is also participating in other trainings asynchronously. Pulling from her understanding of the neurobiology of stress and trauma, she began to look at this situation from a trauma-responsive lens. No one really knew if Ray had a trauma history or not, but Terry remembered from the training that knowing a child's trauma history is not needed to use a trauma-responsive approach. She assumed that the stress teachers were experiencing from these interactions with Ray—and his continual verbal threats to their physical and emotional safety—were leading them to become more reactive and likely approaching Ray, his family and their disciplinary practices in a reactive way (from their lower brainstem). She realized it was critical for her, as the site supervisor, to create an opportunity to slow things down and to talk with the teachers and then separately, with Ray's parents. Terry scheduled one meeting with the teachers and a separate one with Ray's mother and father. She also observed Ray throughout the week in different contexts including outdoors, indoors, during free play, in transitions throughout the day and both at structured and unstructured times. Terry took notes during all of her observations to record, without judgment or evaluation, what she was seeing in Ray's behavior throughout the day (drop-off/pick up, free play, transition, small group, outdoor, lunch, circle time etc.).

Terry learned a tremendous amount by having the two conversations and completing these observations of Ray. She learned that when Ray was not dysregulated (when he was in a calm state), he was described as sweet, caring and engaged. Terry learned that Ray is a very sensitive child and gets triggered when he feels something is unfair to himself or others. His behavior moves from calm → dysregulated quickly when he receives punitive discipline (shaming, lecturing in front of other children, threats to call a parent), as he moves to dysregulation, he begins to make threats and becomes combative (fight mode). Both Ray's parents and his teachers were very stressed by the patterns that were occurring with Ray at the center and their communication broke down as they began blaming one another. Terry understood—using her new knowledge of state-dependent functioning, that this is what relationships and interactions look like when everyone is operating from the survival or lower parts of their brain and not from their cortex.

Terry decided to call a family-teacher meeting to begin to talk about next steps for Ray. Before that meeting, she had a pre-meeting with her teachers. She knew the importance of using trauma-responsive strategies to help her staff have a safe environment where they could share their concerns without fear of evaluation and/or judgment, where they could experience a felt sense of safety and feel "heard" and validated. During the meeting with her teachers, Terry invited them to talk about their experiences and feelings related to working with Ray and to unload their built-up emotions including their fears and their hopes for resolution. She also led them through a group calming mindfulness activity from an activity book they use. The activity is called Tree Breathing (imagine you're a tree in a windy storm and then a calm sunny day...). Terry knew that creating this time was critical to help her teachers enter the family meeting in a calm and regulated state instead of in a reactive (defensive, accusatory, judgmental) state. The parent meeting was scheduled for a few hours after the staff meeting.

Terry started off the teacher-parent meeting with a strength-based approach and set an expectation of safety for everyone involved. She stated, So, I'm really grateful to all of you for giving your time to participate in this meeting. I want to be really mindful of our time. I believe we all agreed we would finish the meeting by 7pm, is that everyone else's understanding? Let's start by focusing on what we all recognize as Ray's many strengths. Here is what I have personally observed and heard in my conversations with all of you:

◆ Ray has a very strong sense of right and wrong or what he feels is right and wrong. And he acts upon that.
◆ Ray is very protective towards people and those he cares about.
◆ Ray is very sensitive and affectionate and caring about others.
◆ Ray loves helping the other children.
◆ Ray is a very sweet boy and very smart.

After learning there was a common understanding of Ray's strengths, next, Terry invited everyone to share some of their emerging concerns.

◆ If Ray is not doing something right, it makes him mad.
◆ Ray does not like to make mistakes.
◆ When Ray doesn't do something right, he blames himself instead of other people.
◆ Ray becomes dysregulated if things are unjust or wrong or if he is not perfect. A teacher shares, "What that looks like is he fights by hitting, using threating words or raising his voice if he sees another child being treated by a classmate unfairly" (i.e., Taking their toy).
◆ Ray becomes reactive when someone or something lets him down. Mom shares, "If I don't follow through with what I say at home, then he gets let down and shows it by hitting his brother, me or yelling at the person he is angry with."
◆ Ray becomes even more triggered if he is (or perceives he is) punished, shamed or called out in front of others or if someone is mad at him or shares disappointment. He only hears, "I am bad." The Instructional Assistant shared a time that he was hitting another child and she jumped in reactively in front of all the other kids and

said, "We don't hit our friends; you need to use your words." After that, his behavior became more escalated and he made verbal threats to me (e.g., I hate you).

After allowing everyone a chance to share, Terry pauses to summarize the common themes of strengths and concerns. She explains: Based on all the observations that I've personally made, the valuable feedback I learned in our prior conversations and based on what has been shared in today's meeting, we are identifying several common themes. May I share them with you to make sure I got them all right? Terry then writes them on a flip chart and repeats them back verbally. She remembers that when people are in a stressful state, they sometimes need visual cues in addition to auditory cues to help their cortex focus and attend to the information. She also wanted to make sure everyone in the meeting had a felt sense of being heard. She understood that when the limbic part of our brains feel heard, this is a stress-reducing and regulating experience. Terry began, "So, we observe stress behaviors more often when Ray perceives something as unfair. Because he cares so much about people being treated fairly, he will intervene when he believes something is not 'right'." When this happens, it feels to the adults around him that he is doing this in an inappropriate way like yelling at another child or threatening the teachers. When an adult tries to correct his behavior, he perceives even more threat and that is when he shifts into verbal threats that are the most concerning to the staff. Did I get that right? Everyone nodded and agreed unanimously.

Terry then asks, **"Does anyone have anything else to add or are we ready to move to next steps?"** Before brainstorming begins, the Instructional Aide, Shiya, raised her hand. She said she just thought of something. She shares:

One-time Ray was triggered because he was observing one boy being mean to another girl so he went over to fight him. At that moment, I quickly called over to

Ray and asked him to help me with something. When he came over to me we talked privately about what happened. Ray was able to share how he felt and after a few minutes when he had calmed down, I asked if he was open to speaking with Teacher Mindy to find ways to solve the problem without hurting others or even himself. He said he was and later, Teacher Mindy said this strategy was really effective with Ray.

Terry thanked Shiya for sharing this story and there was a unanimous agreement that talking to Ray privately should be added to the list of strategies and next steps.

As the meeting came close to the end, the site supervisor summarized what was shared as common strengths and concerns and the teachers and parents acknowledged they were in agreement. Each person was asked if they wanted to add any additional information. They proceeded together to move on to concrete next steps...

◆ Ray's teachers would work on remaining calm when he is activated as everyone agreed that Ray does much better if his teachers are not dysregulated (in their language or nonverbal behavior).
◆ When Ray was triggered, his teachers would find ways to talk to him privately, but they would always start with listening to him first to help him calm his stress response system so he could access his cortex in order to engage in problem solving (calm the downstairs brain first before connecting him to the cortex/upstairs for solutions and problem solving).
◆ In the classroom and at home, Ray's teachers and parents would help him learn how to identify his feelings to help Ray build a vocabulary and way to communicate verbally and non-verbally what he is feeling. The site supervisor would schedule time with the teachers and parents to come up with a more specific plan and next steps to implement emotional literacy strategies.

♦ The teachers would begin to teach Ray and the other children in the class some self-regulation strategies that they could use when they feel their sensations or emotions rise up and they need to find ways to calm their body to feel safe (e.g., breathing, asking an adult for help, creating a safe place in the classroom to get).

♦ They would schedule another meeting in a month to check back in.

♦ Terry extended an offer that they all could call her throughout the week and outside of these scheduled meetings for anything.

Reflective/Discussion Questions

♦ Do you have a child whose behavior frightens you and have you found yourself moving more toward your downstairs, more reactive part of your brain with this child and/or family?

♦ When you were triggered by a child's behavior, did you find yourself focusing on the challenging behavior but forgetting to look past the behavior to the meaning behind the child's behavior? (Is the child trying to gain someone or something, avoid someone or something, express a sensation/emotion or is the child telling us they feel unsafe in the moment?)

♦ What sensations did you feel in your body (i.e., head, throat, breathing neck, stomach, heart, hands, legs, feet)? What feelings did you have (i.e., angry, hurt, scared, sad, frustrated)?

♦ Was there a situation where you used some of the following trauma-responsive strategies:
  • Slowing things down (Understanding Stress and Trauma)
  • Using reflective questions to help people name how they feel to calm their big emotions (Understand Stress and Trauma, Establishing Safety and Predictability

and Promoting Coping, Resilience, Healing and Wellness)

- Looking behind the challenging behavior to what story the child is trying to communicate with their behavior (Understanding Stress and Trauma)
- Identifying strengths in addition to concerns (Focus on Strengths and Assets)
- Thinking of when the challenging behavior did not occur and why? (Focus on Strengths and Assets)
- Identifying triggers for the adult and for the child (Understanding Stress and Trauma)
- Asking permission to move on during meetings (Provide Opportunities for Agency and Control)
- Summarizing and checking for understanding in a meeting (Creating Power Sharing Partnerships, Provide Opportunities for Agency and Control)
- Giving everyone a shared voice in a meeting (Creating Power Sharing Partnerships, Provide Opportunities for Agency and Control)

◆ Case Study #5: "The Struggle Is Real: What Does It Mean for Me to Be a Trauma-Responsive District Level Administrator with Multiple Intersecting Dilemmas?"—Ming Lau, Preschool and Elementary Program Coordinator, Department of Special Education

I am a program coordinator for the department of special education at a public school district. I oversee special education programs, supervise and evaluate a group of teachers, paraeducators, specialists, such as the behaviorists and the occupational therapists. And I also oversee program managers. I attend high-profile IEP meetings and oftentimes I represent the district's interests. I find myself the target of parents' and teachers' anger, frustration, exasperations and deep hurt. Parents tell me that I have harmed their children by not giving them, from their perspective, what their child deserves. Teachers tell me the "District" is not supportive of their work and demands too much (paperwork, curriculum, initiatives, etc.). A big part of my job is to hire special education (SPED) teachers, yet the burnout rate for SPED teachers is high. What are the factors that lead our teachers to leave? I have learned that one important factor is whether we, as supervising administrators, have enough finesse to create a buffer between the constant demands from the county, the state and the federal government and our teachers. I am continually in conversations with my colleagues about how to safeguard our teachers from the stressors of their daily job.

Another reason our teachers leave their positions is because of a stressful experience they have with a family. Many of our families' needs are significant and families might direct their intense emotions, including anger and grief, towards our teachers. They might blame teachers when their children are not progressing faster or because their child's teacher has not "fixed" their children's developmental challenges and/or special needs. I remember one parent who threatened me and my staff. He very angrily told us that we had one more year to ensure that his child had progressed enough to move out of special education and be placed within a general education classroom. Unfortunately, this was not immediately possible for his son because of a combined intellectual disability and autism. In addition, because of a misgiving of the public school system, the family had kept the child from attending school for a whole year. We were witness to his feelings of intense sadness, anger and the grieving he was doing in coming to terms with his child's special needs. This can be a common experience for SPED teachers and can feel stressful when these emotions are combined with verbal and/or physical threats by a parent or family member. I have had staff who needed to begin therapy after really challenging interactions with a family. Cumulative stressful and traumatic experiences like these wear down our teachers. And me too as their administrator.

On top of managing these difficult situations, I also have to contend with what I experience as discrimination based on my gender, race and ethnicity. I often feel that because I am not White, many families and even our upper management team do not give much weight to my recommendations and my opinions. There are families who would rather talk to my supervisor, who is White, because they tell me, she would better understand their needs and be more effective in allocating resources to support their child. I've also been told that I should be removed from a case with a Black family because I am not Black and therefore, could not be as effective in managing their case. When families of color share their displeasure at meetings that they do not see any administrators of color, I wonder what color they see when they look at me. I am an Asian American woman who was an immigrant to this country. I am bicultural and bilingual, a first-generation college attendee and a college graduate. Yet, families and supervisors don't see these things when they look at me.

Being a trauma-responsive administrator for early childhood special education services is extremely complex and a daily struggle. Taking a trauma-responsive approach begins by focusing on building trusting relationships with others. Special Education is a legal minefield where services and time are given a dollar amount to be negotiated between lawyers and families It can be very inequitable as some parents have social capital and financial means to get more resources. They know the system, they know where to find a lawyer who specializes in special education and they can pay for an advocate to argue and demand more for their child.

Building trust with my staff means helping them feel safe and supported. Building trust with parents and families means identifying individualized supports for their children that allow us to meet the legal requirements of what they are entitled to but also realistically align with the limited resources we have available in our district. It also means in some cases, helping parents and families move through a grieving process of accepting their child's developmental disability or special need. And building trust within my institution and school district is perhaps the biggest struggle of all. You cannot build trust until you are *seen* by those around you. To be invisibilized is to sow the seeds of distrust. What does it mean for me to be a trauma-responsive district level administrator? I don't have an easy answer even for myself. I have many conflicting identities when it comes to thinking about myself as an administrator.

Becoming trauma-responsive is not easy and it's not always straightforward as Ming Lau highlights when you have staff and families with varying and complex needs, you are in a position of leadership that is highly demanding and you experience racism on a daily basis and don't feel respected, supported and/or visible in your workplace. This chronic toxic stress will make it harder to do trauma-responsive work with others and it might adversely impact you over the long term emotionally, socially and/or physically. For some people, this might require making a choice to change jobs to stop your own suffering so you have the capacity to be present with others. For others who can't or choose not to leave their positions, it will be more important than ever to build in ways to care for yourself and re-charge your energy outside of work and to the extent you can, during work.

Reflection/Discussion Questions

High chronic stress can adversely impact health and well-being (physically, emotionally and socially) and prevents us from having the ability to have the restored energy reserves to support families and to face daily adversities without being triggered into reactive parts of our brain. When your workplace comes with high levels of stress:

- ◆ What small ways do you buffer your stress and promote health, restoration and wellness for yourself at work and/or outside of work? For others? If you are a leader or supervisor, for the staff you supervise?
- ◆ As Ming Lau's story highlights, experiencing racism and micro-aggressions, not being acknowledged as having credible or valued expertise and feeling misunderstood, mischaracterized and invisible in the workplace on a continual basis creates the conditions for toxic stress and trauma—e.g., perceptions of fear, lack of agency and control or hopelessness. How much of Ming Lau's experience rings true for you? If you have any of these experiences in your workplace, do you recognize when it happens, how it makes you feel and the impact it has on your body and on your emotions?
- ◆ How do you cope so that this stress does not adversely impact you socially, emotionally or physically? Are there culturally responsive strategies (see Nicholson, Driscoll, Kurtz, Wesley & Benitez, 2020) you use to cope, buffer the stress or trauma to protect yourself from the adverse effects of this cumulative stress?

◆ Case Study #6: "I Feel You. I Hear You"—Muriel Johnson, Lead Preschool Teacher, Private Preschool

We had an adorable boy in our program. His mom was biracial and dad was Black, from Tennessee. Mom made the decision to enroll him at our school but wanted dad to see the school so he scheduled a visit. He happened to come on a day where all the kids were running around in their underwear doing water play. And I could just see the look on his face, "Like, oh, hell no!" I could tell he was just like, "I don't know what his mother has done, but there's no way that my son is going to be running around in his underwear with all these little White kids. It's just wrong and he's southern." I said, "Michael, it looks like you have some questions or some thoughts going on." He was very polite and responded, "Well actually I do." I reassured him, "I'm available if you want to talk or run something by me." And so he asked, "Do they always be running around like this?" "Yeah. In the summer-time, they do." He said, "Oh, I can't. I just can't. I'm from the South. I can't ..." I said, **"I feel you. I hear you."**

Then he said, "Well, if my son attends here, he's not going to be allowed to do that." I shared, "Well, you have a right to, you're his parent, but we're not going to enforce that." We're not going to let all these kids run around and be free and then deny him of this experience. So, if you tell him, 'Don't take your clothes off,' and he decides that he wants to run around in his underwear with the other kids, we're not going to make him put his clothes on. I'm just letting you know upfront because that would be against our ethics of kids getting to be free and have this experience."

He thought for a moment and then asked, "Well, why do you all let them do this?" I responded, "Well, tell me ... so, you grew up in the South. What was the most fun thing that you got to do when you were a kid?" He started talking about working in the fields with his grandfather and running around. I said, "What about times when it was really hot?" He explained that his grandma would make lemonade. And so I said, "That must have just felt so good. Oh yes, you're smiling as you're reminiscing about your experience being a child in the South." I asked, "Did you go barefoot sometimes?" He's said, "Yeah, I did. I went barefoot." So then I told him, "Well, that feeling that you're describing is what we allow the kids to have here. Look at them. I saw that you were kind of appalled, but do you see their faces? And do you hear them? They are getting to have some freedom in a safe environment. I respect whatever you want to do with your son, but I'm just letting you know that if he's here, we cannot promise you that we're going to make sure he doesn't take off his clothes." And he responded, "Okay, I respect that. I got it."

I didn't think they would be returning to the school. But they did and their little boy did get to run free and dad became my buddy. And yet, we have some staff in our program who rolled their eyes when talking about this dad, "Oh, my gosh, Michael doesn't want his kid … that is so ridiculous!" Their attitude was discounting this father's feelings and not attempting to understand his cultural perspective. They were being disrespectful in so many ways and their words were communicating, "We're superior. We're early childhood educators. We know what's best, and these parents are so ignorant. Can you believe that he's upset about that?" But they never even considered or tried to learn the perspective of the parent. When I see my colleagues complaining about and criticizing parents I always suggest, "Let's think about where they're coming from" so we can build empathy for them. Our first reaction is far too often to discount parents' and families' perspectives."

Muriel shows us that family engagement does not mean that we listen to parents, take their lead and always do everything they say. It also means using our expert knowledge of child development. When listening to parents, we can often land on different pathways in decision-making:

◆ Listen, take in their perspective and jump to their side
◆ Listen, compromise on a solution between your expertise and theirs
◆ Listen, respectfully communicate the differing views and share the "why" behind your decision

Muriel had a difficult conversation, but it included respecting the voice of the parent, listening to how he felt, respecting his words, thoughts and reactions while at the same time exploring new ways of knowing and understanding young children's development. She approaches the conversation using the trauma-responsive principle, Building Mutually Respectful and Trusting Relationships.

Reflection/Discussion Questions

- ◆ How did Muriel make a connection with this father?
- ◆ Even in a conversation where initially two people disagree, how did Muriel still maintain a mutually respectful and trusting interaction with dad?
- ◆ Have you had a difficult conversation like this in the past where you and a parent had differing views? Can you think of the following as you reflect on that conversation…
  - • Did you take the time to listen to how the parent felt, and to learn about and try to understand their thoughts, feelings and reactions?
  - • How did you both come to a final decision? Did you agree to disagree, shift to their perspective or come to a compromise? Did the relationship continue with mutual respect and trust following this conversation? How do you know and what signs lead you to believe there was still trust?
- ◆ How can you use questions like Muriel did to create a pause, to slow things down and to center the parent or family member's voice in an interaction and then to deeply listen and be responsive to what you hear?

References

Nicholson, J., Driscoll, P., Kurtz, J., Wesley, L., & Benitez, D. (2020). Culturally responsive self-care practices for early childhood educators. New York, NY: Routledge.

Conclusion

Throughout this book we have shared a range of Trauma-Responsive and Resilience-Building principles and concrete strategies to guide your work in creating a robust family engagement approach within your program, school or agency. We recognize that each family is unique with their own history, culture, sources of stress, trauma, coping skills, resilience factors and approaches to healing. No two families are alike, and a strategy that works with one family may not with another. This book is not intended to be a one size fits all. In fact, one successful family engagement strategy might not be the best approach with another family. Responsive family engagement is not a recipe early childhood professionals can take away and apply equally to every family. Although family engagement is not a mathematical formula, it is based in the science of human connection, learning, engagement and resilience/healing.

Many people incorrectly assume that when people alter their beliefs, changes in behavior will follow. However, many research studies document that changing conscious beliefs and intentions does not necessarily lead people to change their behavior, especially if the goal is long-term sustained behavior change. As a result, we offer some suggestions drawn from research describing the factors that support adults to start new and desired habits (e.g., using regulation strategies to maintain calm and support

DOI: 10.4324/9781003127666-12

self-care) and to "unlearn" and disrupt unwanted and harmful habits (e.g., deficit language and thinking about families):

To Learn a New/Desired Habit (mindset, behavior or practice): **The goal is "Autopilot"**

The key is to teach your brain to associate this new habit (e.g., taking deep breaths to stay regulated, treating families like an "invited guest," asking a question to invite families' voices into a conversation) with your daily interactions. Make it seamlessly woven into what you do in your work by doing the following things (Wood, 2019):

When doing something is effortless = lower friction

◆ **Make it easy.** This is absolutely critical. Start small with a strategy you can integrate into what you are already doing. To use breathing for regulation, open staff meetings with a collective deep breath. Reduce the difficulty, effort or what researchers call "friction" associated with the new habit. We represent this with the metaphor of a slide: Children don't need to work hard to go down a slide. There is little friction (effort, challenge) and once they sit down, gravity does the work. Similarly, you are more likely to build a new habit if you make it as easy

Starting a Desired Habit
(Mindset + Behavior)

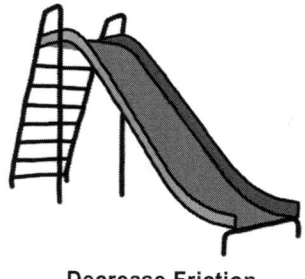

Decrease Friction

FIGURE 11.1
Slide
Alice Blecker

as possible to fit into your routines and current practice (reduce the friction). We encourage you to take small and realistic actions steps—what Zaretta Hammond (2015) describes as "bite size actions"—that allow you to work for change in realistic and accessible ways. If the change is too complex or difficult, chances are less likely you will stick with it.

◆ **Repeat it often.** The goal is to make the new habit become unconscious and therefore, automatic (on "autopilot"). Structure your environment to make it easy to auto-mate or practice the desired habit frequently (e.g., each time you see a family, share one positive observation of their child from that day versus only doing so at formal meeting times or building in regulation breaks at the same time every day). By doing this, you open up brain capacity for the cortex as the new habit does not require cognitive effort and attention.

◆ **Identify the immediate reward.** We are much more likely to build new habits when they are associated in our brains with some type of reward. Rewards associated with the implementation of trauma-responsive practices could be increased feelings of safety, calm, joy or pride, having small wins and progress acknowledged in staff meetings, reducing stress through organizational care routines and support from colleagues, or feeling "heard" in a conversation with a supervisor. Having to wait for a reward months or years away is much less likely to inspire people to change their behavior.

Neurons Wire Together, If They Fire Together

For a behavior to become a habit, it needs to be performed frequently and repeated many times over to rewire the brain. This principle is known as the Hebbian learning rule: "If interconnected neurons become active very close in time during a particular event, their connection strengthens and 'a memory' of this event is formed. In other words, 'neurons wire together, if they fire together' " (Krupic, 2017).

To Unlearn and Disrupt an Unwanted or Harmful Habit (mindset, behavior or practice): **The goal is "Increasing Awareness"** (Wood, 2019)

When doing something requires effort = higher friction

◆ **To unlearn or interrupt a bad habit, try to make yourself just a little bit more conscious of it.** The idea is to make a small change in your practice that increases your awareness of the unwanted habit and requires you to think about it momentarily. In other words, you slightly increase the level of friction—making it just a bit more challenging or effortful to engage in the habit you want to unlearn. We use the image of a playground rock wall to represent the idea of increasing friction. For most children, climbing up a rock wall requires a bit more cognitive effort and attention than going down a slide.

Increasing the level of friction might include: learning to stop and notice the language you are using to describe a family (am I focusing on their strengths or deficits?), or learning to pause

Ending an Undesired Habit
(Mindset + Behavior)

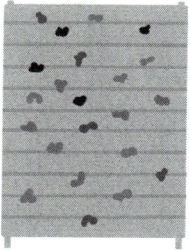

Increase Friction

FIGURE 11.2
Rock wall
Alice Blecker

and do a body scan to notice if/when your stress response system has been activated, or learning to ask a question to pause your reactivity in a conversation ("I heard you say Jason doesn't feel safe here, can you tell me a bit more about that?"). Making the unwanted habit just a little more conscious allows you to you stop, think and make important discoveries that can lead to re-centering attention on your values and the "why" inspiring the work you do. ("Oh this is not what I intended. This is not aligned with my values and the way I want to show up for children and families. I can make a different choice and do better.")

◆ **Modify the environment to de-incentivize the habit.** Think of ways to make changes in your program or practice that will make it harder to engage in the habit (increase friction). Think of this like putting guard rails in place. One example is seen with programs that are creating procedures that make it much harder to suspend or expel young children as they require many steps in a process that allow staff to disrupt harmful disciplinary practices. We saw another example in Chapter 4 where parents and families' stress related behaviors are being reframed as reflecting their passion and deep care for their child. By learning to stop their reactivity and ask a question, "Where is there passion here?" one program is working to ensure that deficit stories are not told about families. Instead, this question shifts them into a strength-based approach that acknowledges that these behaviors are stories that families communicate--based in their love and concern for their children—about how they feel and what they need.

Both of these strategies will help you shift out of "auto-pilot" and bring your attention to the undesired attitude, belief, behavior or practice and give you a chance to decide if you want to change it. This is the heart of continuous learning that becomes the foundation of transformative change.

It is easy to become overwhelmed with all of the suggestions and ideas outlined in this book. The most important thing you can do to get started is to make sure you are clear about your "why" for wanting to strengthen and improve your work with families as this will be your guidepost every single day. Be patient with yourself. Give yourself and others grace as you continue on your learning journey and know that building new habits takes time. Every day that you embrace trauma-responsive language, mindsets, behaviors and practices in your work with families, you will not only positively impact the current families you serve, but also create ripples of influence for future generations.

A simple reminder as we close our book: *Every dose of positive relational connection you provide to parents and families in everyday interactions is equivalent to a therapeutic encounter* (Perry, 2017). Over time, these encounters have tremendous power to buffer experiences of stress and trauma, support healing and strengthen well-being and thrivance for children and adults.

References

Hammond, Z. (2015). *Culturally responsive teaching and the brain. Promoting authentic engagement and rigor among culturally and linguistically diverse students.* Thousand Oaks, CA: Corwin.

Krupic, J. (2017). Wire together, fire apart. *Science, 357*(6355), 974–975. doi: 10.1126/science.aao4159.

Perry, B. (2017). *The boy who was raised as a dog and other stories from a child psychiatrist's notebook. What traumatized children can teach us about loss, love and healing.* New York, NY: Basic Books.

Wood, W. (2019). *Good habits, bad habits: The science of making positive changes that stick.* New York, NY: Farrar, Straus and Giroux.

Resources

The Harvard Family Research Project www.hfrp.org This website describes the benefits of family engagement and the connections across educational organizations, nationally and globally. Includes videos and resources for early childhood schools, community-based programs, libraries and after schoo. programs.

Strengthening Families™ Protective Factors framework, Center for the Study of Social Policy https://cssp.org/wp-content/uploads/2018/11/About-StrengtheningFamilies.pdf Site describes the five protective factors for families, programs and communities.

The Head Start Parent, Family, and Community Engagement Interactive Framework http://eclkc.ohs.acf.hhs.gov/hslc/tta-system/family/framework A road map that can be used in program-wide strategic planning, program design and management, continuous learning and improvement activities, as well as with governing bodies and parent groups. Website includes research, resources, and regulations related to program foundations, program impact areas, family engagement outcomes, and child outcomes. Also see the following Guide to Developing

Relationships with Families: https://eclkc.ohs.acf.hhs.gov/sites/default/files/pdf/building-partnerships-developing-relationships-families.pdf

The U.S. Department of Education's, Partners in Education A Dual Capacity-Building Framework for Family–School Partnerships www2.ed.gov/documents/family-community/partners-education.pdf Downloadable resource about integrating family engagement strategies as an integral part of education reform efforts. Based on research demonstrating the beneficial effects of parental involvement and family-school partnerships and that "parent and community ties" can have a systemic and sustained effect on learning outcomes for children and on whole school improvement when combined with other essential supports.

National Center on Parent, Family and Community Engagement (NCPFCE) https://startearly.org/post/start-early-chosen-to-lead-implementation-national-center-for-parent-family-community-engagement/ The NCPFCE identifies, develops and disseminates evidence-based best practices to support the growth and development of young children and strengthen families and communities. Its work includes providing training and technical assistance on staff-family relationship building practices that are culturally and linguistically responsive; integrated and systemic family engagement strategies that are outcomes-based; and consumer education, family leadership, family economic stability, and individualized support for families facing adversity. They strive to bring family engagement, parent voice and community engagement to the forefront of early childhood education.

A Note About the Cover

The River Metaphor as a Symbolic Representation of the Complex and Essential Relationship between Early Childhood Professionals and Families. We include the image of a river on the cover to represent the critical role of parents and families in the lives of young children. This image also represents the need for trauma-responsive, resilience-building and healing-centered approaches to collaboration and partnership with families in early childhood programs and services. Why use a river metaphor?

Rivers are diverse, powerful, dynamic and beautiful. Rivers are diverse and have their own distinctive and inherent beauty. They flow at varying speeds, elevations and through vastly diverse landscapes and climates throughout the world. The energy and power of a river is significant and responsible for driving change—whether still pools, gentle ripples or fast-moving rapids, running down mountains, over cliffs or through green valleys, a river is dynamic with power to shape the landscape all around it. Rivers are a valuable resource that supply energy and create and sustain life for many organisms, animals, plants and communities. In fact, rivers are often at the center of villages, towns, cities and communities.

This is similar to the early childhood field where families come with different histories, values, perceptions, beliefs,

temperaments, ways of knowing, strengths, vulnerabilities and lived experiences. These factors and others
influence what they bring into and how they influence
our early childhood programs, policies and practices if
we are committed to sharing power and agency with
them—listening to their ideas, partnering with them in
decision-making and remaining flexible and responsive
to their changing needs and input that can create new and
expanded opportunities for our growth as professionals
in supporting children to thrive in our care. Just like the
interdependent relationships between a river and the
surrounding environment, our early childhood programs
can become deeply responsive and engaged with the
parents and families and communities we serve. We can
co-create environments where there is a sense of community, belonging, and where there are critical supports and
resources in times of need—from basic needs including
food, clothing and diapers to support groups, discussions
about children's development and/or mental health
services.

**Rivers encounter many obstacles that prevent or limit
their capacity to flow.** Rivers do not choose their course but
instead, are constrained by the unique and dynamic conditions
of the surrounding environment. Although they encounter many
obstacles that temporarily slow down or disrupt their flow,
with the exception of dams, river water—pulled by the force of
gravity—will continue flowing using new pathways that adjust
and navigate around these barriers.

Just like the river must navigate risk factors, so is the field
of early childhood education. Working with families who
have experienced stress, inequities, trauma or historical
trauma can create obstacles and barriers but ultimately,
like the river, families contain within them resilience
factors and an inherent movement toward health and
healing. If we provide trauma-responsive programs
we can disrupt inequities, offer families support, create

partnerships and interactions that buffer stress, and partner with them to navigate the barriers (adversities) they face despite the challenges and burdens they experience as they are parenting young children.

The health of the river is significantly impacted by the health (or lack thereof) of the environment around it. Rivers and their health or fragility are highly contingent upon the larger ecosystems they exist within. When actions are taken to intentionally maintain the health of the ecosystem (policies and practices that sustain clean water, air, soil, and reduce overfishing/illegal fishing, environmental pollution etc.), the river will thrive and generate and support an abundance of life forms. If instead, the surrounding environment erodes from compounding threats that destabilize the health of the ecosystem (climate change, deforestation), the river will mirror these conditions and become increasingly fragile and unable to support or sustain life.

Parents and families are deeply impacted by the larger society in which they live and their access to resources and supports that support their health, stability and well-being. The more inequity in a society—where only certain children and families have access to quality health care, education, food, employment, financial stability, etc., and others are oppressed or "held down" and denied access to opportunities and resources—the more marginalized families will experience toxic stress and trauma.

The fluid and dynamic river is a symbol of our individual and collective learning journeys. Water reflects flexibility and the state of embracing change. It will always take the form in which it is held but it can also carve out mountains and rock to make its way through and continue forward. Below the surface of the water there is an ecosystem that is layered with life-giving resources and threats. Universally, and for centuries in cultures around the world, water has been seen as a symbol of life, renewal, healing and transformation.

Shifting to a trauma-responsive family engagement approach with diverse parents and families will require humility, continuous listening and learning, a willingness to take risks and experience vulnerability for early childhood professionals. The power for water to impact the environment but to also mirror the environment attributes in which it is given is similar to working with families. Families in their own right have power to carve out their own beautiful lives <u>and</u> like the river, they are impacted by the environments in which they interact (schools, systems, services, social supports). Water reminds us to dive beneath the surface of our feelings and use intuition to better understand ourselves and families. This symbol helps us see that things are never as they seem at the surface. When working with families, we are reminded by the water to always look beyond the surface to the depth of acknowledging our histories, our stressors and trauma, our resilience, strengths, skills, feelings and lived experiences that help ourselves and families to cope, heal and thrive and that give meaning to mindsets and behaviors. As adults, we remember that we have a unique reservoir of knowledge that exists within us all and that we are ALL in constant momentum toward growth and healing.

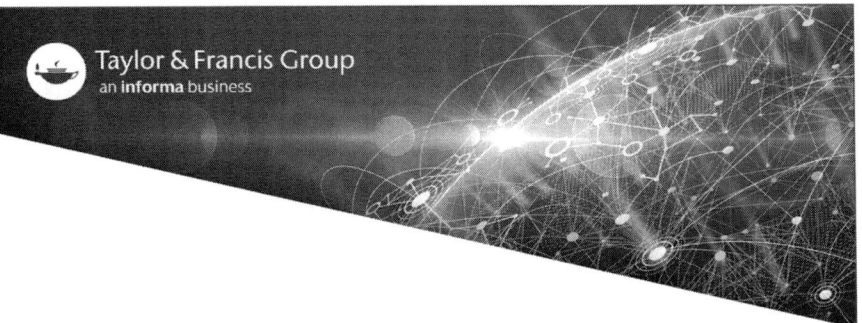
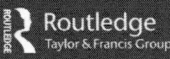
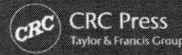

Printed in the United States
by Baker & Taylor Publisher Services